Sassafras Street

Human Connection Through the Eyes of Caregivers

Diane Wintz, MD, FACS
Kelly Wright, MSN

SASSAFRAS STREET

HUMAN CONNECTION THROUGH THE EYES OF CAREGIVERS

ISBN: 979-8-218-84703-6 (Print)
ISBN: 979-8-218-84704-3 (E-Book)

Cover Imagery: Design created using Canva Pro art on September 19, 2025, by Melissa Karren.

Contents

Introduction

Sassafras is a plant with medicinal properties. It is often used as a tea and can be therapeutic or harmful based on the dose. It is a yin-yang treatment, both a positive and a negative, running parallel to the emotion required for the practice of medicine; a roller coaster of failure, success, surprise, disappointment, anxiety, and relief which patients and families are free to feel but which health-care providers must temper and control.

SASSAFRAS, A NATIVE TREE on Galveston Bay in Texas, was the namesake for an ice cream parlor on the coast. The shop was located on the old boardwalk of that beach town, a short street lined with unique shops and cafés.

The wind was warm coming off the water, and I felt the scratchy sand embedded in my shoes as my grandmother led me into the shop. I was a five-year-old child in a literal candy store, and the world was my oyster. A multicolored array of candy sticks was displayed on the far wall, showcasing all of the different flavors. My grandmother nudged me to grab a few that I wanted. The biggest decision of my life took center stage: which sticks to choose. The brightly colored purple, turquoise, yellow, green, and pink were not my favorite flavors, but they looked so pretty when held together—like a rainbow. My favorite flavor—sassafras (or root beer)—was brown, which didn't match the others. It wouldn't be admired by anyone, and I couldn't show it off, but I would certainly enjoy eating it. If I chose an assortment of sticks in beautiful colors, the girls in my class would be excited to pick theirs. None of them wanted a brown stick, even if it was candy.

My grandmother, arguably the most impatient person walking the planet at that time, tapped her shoe and told me to hurry it up. The sassafras sticks were placed in a paper bag, concealed.

We sat at a high-top table and ate ice cream as she began the age-old game of discussing my career aspirations. She explained in great detail why I should become a doctor. "Don't you want to be smart? Don't you want to be important? Don't you want to fix people and have them admire you?"

This line of questioning morphed into expectations for straight A's and a focus on science and math, with her providing constant examples of why medicine should be my chosen field. She got my parents on this same bandwagon, so I heard the same messaging time and again. "You can do anything, and with your brain, you should."

I went through school dedicated, but it was always a stressor. And despite the encouragement, I didn't have a definitive goal or direction other than to do well. It wasn't until I finished my first year of college that I determined I would try to be a doctor.

My grandmother was an incredible powerhouse. As the family matriarch, she knew everything. She was intelligent and articulate, a natural leader, a bit bossy, and absolutely amazing. I spent most of my childhood weekends with her, and we consistently followed her favorite Saturday pattern of groceries, lunch, and shopping followed by laundry and dinner with the family.

As a very young girl, I saw my grandmother working, which was unusual for grandmothers at the time. She had a job at a dentist's office as a bookkeeper. There was a disruptive financial strain within the business that threatened her position, but she determined to make herself invaluable to her boss. Within about a week, she moved stocks and investments, made a significant profit, and proved that she was essential to the entire enterprise, which was just one office at the time.

They eventually grew to oversee thirteen incorporated offices, with my grandmother serving as their senior vice president. I witnessed all of this before I was ten, and it had a profound influence on me, instilling the belief that anything was possible. I grew up believing that I could achieve anything I wanted to do. The world was my oyster, open for the taking. I still carry that belief with me today, confident that I can accomplish anything my heart and mind may conceive. My grandmother was instrumental in showing me that tangible goals are born from unattainable dreams. She also would have been proud to see that her two decades of coaching paid off.

I became a physician. I am currently the chief of trauma surgery. I spent my residency and fellowship training learning the intricacies of providing care to injured or emergent surgical patients. These patients were generally young and had been injured in high-energy mechanisms.

Over the past several years, the geriatric population has grown, consistent with the number of baby boomers who are aging. My own practice of medicine evolved due to the changing population patterns. My interest suddenly shifted to providing care for older adults. It was a new challenge for me: managing the underlying diseases, talking about issues related to end-of-life, addressing changing levels of independence, and putting the medical care into the context of each patient's goals for self. Patients sixty-five and older now encompass one-third of my practice. Their care needs are interesting, and often the decision-making is complex, which appeals to me. I can't help but wonder if that is my grandmother's nudge continuing from beyond.

In 2018, there was one patient who impacted my perspective, and based on his experience in my care, I wanted to make a change. He was eighty years old and living independently. He had fallen down in his home, where he had lain on the ground injured until someone had found him. He was eventually tended to by emergency medical services (EMS) and brought to the hospital where my team took over. We stood over him and went through the motions of examining, taking vitals, and collecting his belongings for safekeeping. He was found to have a brain injury and was admitted for ongoing monitoring and treatment. The whole process was routine.

The next morning, I went to visit him, and his nurse stopped me outside his room. She intimated that he was delirious. She described him hearing and seeing things that were not real. So I went into the room, and I said, "Your nurse tells me that you are confused."

He looked right at me, and he said, "I am not confused. I was attacked by a gang last night."

He began to describe his experience. He was amnesic due to his fall, but he knew he had been helped off the ground by medics and had been brought to a hospital. He remembered that he had been surrounded by a group of people in the emergency department who had all pulled on him and screamed at him. His phone and belongings were missing, and he didn't have any phone numbers memorized, so he couldn't call anyone for help. He showed me his wrists, which had soft restraints on them. His nurse had applied them for his safety, but to him, they were tying him to the bed and restricting his movement. The lights had been left on all night, and people had come in and out of the room, preventing him from sleeping. Any time he tried to ask a question or demand his belongings, he was shushed, medicated, patted, or told that everything was fine. Things were clearly *not* fine.

In that moment, I was struck by the contrast of our guidelines and system of intake versus his lived experience. We completed our regular therapeutics and monitoring. We certainly were not intending to scare him. I had always been proud of each of my team members, and our complication rates were low. But what he was saying made me realize that there was no consideration for *him* during those initial urgent minutes. It was clear that we hadn't adequately explained our process or listened to him or his concerns.

He further recalled that it must have been a gang because everyone wore matching blue uniforms. I looked down at my navy blue scrubs with a pit in my stomach. This man wasn't delirious, and he wasn't imagining anything. I knew things had to change. If patients perceived our efforts to manage their injuries as gang attacks, we needed to find a different approach. It was the push-pull of sassafras: believing everything was going well because of the effort put in, while missing the inadequacies of the care plans.

So I formed a team with an emphasis on compassionate care for older patients. I wanted to concentrate on the whole person—not just the illness or injury, but the pieces of life that mattered. That program grew and eventually was branded as Generational Health, which was supported by philanthropy.[1]

Our team developed Generational Health from the ground up based on our experience in caring for people in our community. We started with a small pilot program on trauma, a single unit with eighty-three patients enrolled in the program to show results. We had no idea at that time whether the program would be sustainable, durable, or useful. It took several months to prove that a program focusing on strength and cognition during hospitalization led to improved outcomes such as reduced delirium and faster time to homebound discharge. Patients provided feedback and staff continued to modify the program to meet their needs. We later solidified this program for all patients sixty-five and older and added specific pathways to include a geriatric accredited emergency department,[2] age-friendly care or healthy aging,[3] geriatric surgery,[4] and Advanced Illness Management.[5]

The program was expanding and was at a point where it could run regardless of whether I was at work. It happened on a random Thursday that I was sitting with the program manager, Kelly, piling a chip with fresh guacamole while she was asking if we should have a legacy event. We morphed the idea into an initiative to collect stories from the people on our team.

The whole thing was Kelly's idea. The event focused on health-care providers sharing their histories, why they cared, who inspired them, and why community mattered. We thought these stories would be inspiring for anyone going through medical training, for caregivers, and for patients who were facing new challenges in their lives. In our experiences of caring for others and providing self-care, it was often soul-supporting to read or hear about stories of other people who had dealt with something like the challenges we faced.

We had an incredible response from many influential people who later contributed their stories to this book. I tear up even now when I read about Stef's dad, Ari's euloGigi, and Gil's first volunteer experience. These stories were the heart and soul of Generational Health, a health-care program designed by real people for their community. In addition to the many years of training and preparation that went into becoming a health-care professional was the person who had a family, needed a friend, or had gone through loss themselves, who knew what it felt like to be a caregiver to a stranger or a family member, who had health-care expertise balanced with human emotions and heart.

As I started to put this book together, I realized that it needed more of me in it. It wasn't fair to tell everyone else's story and not my own. Where did I fit in? I had been the medical director for the Generational Health program since its inception when it was a tiny pilot program on a single trauma unit before it spread to the general inpatient population at the hospital. Generational Health focused on geriatric care in the acute setting by prioritizing what mattered most to patients. The program was my passion realized, something I'd put my time and energy into creating based on my experience with one patient who had pointed out the ways in which the care had gone awry. For me, it was a full circle of giving and taking, creating Generational Health and providing care that mattered to others, learning and teaching based on professional and personal experience.

I thought a bit about time. How much time I had missed while in school and while training, how much time was required to care for the hospitalized patients, how many nights I spent awake while ruminating on a patient's chart or thinking about a case. How many incredible memories I had of successes. How many miracles I had been able to witness, how many lives had been made better by the medical team, and how many families had more time with their loved ones because of the care that had been applied. Time is the most valuable resource; it is something that can't be replicated, can never be refunded, and only comes around once. The practice of medicine represented the most selfless use of time: true, altruistic giving provided with care and attention, without judgment or expectation of gratitude. I thought about the times when I hadn't been successful in saving someone, when I felt like I had failed at my one job as a surgeon. The internalization of those failures was insurmountable. And I thought about how much time I'd spent going back to those failures and recounting every detail.

I wrote this book to legitimize my time over the past twenty-three years. The dinners where I fell asleep, the birthdays I missed, the family get-togethers I spent studying note cards under the table, every time I walked into a patient's room and wished I could trade places with them for a few hours in a bed—all given the much-deserved respect to my time and what that meant to me to be able to give it to others rather than to myself.

By 2022, the COVID-19 pandemic was winding down, and many of my senior colleagues had made the decision to retire or transition out of medicine altogether. There was an uprising of negativity on social media, often featuring health-care providers in compromising situations. The reality was that the cases were beyond difficult, taxed my emotions, and required complex decision-making. I took the cases home more than I used to. How could I take a break or relax when patients in the intensive care unit (ICU) were fighting for their lives?

I recognized these feelings as burnout, but it was unexpected. There had been plenty of times when I'd felt exhausted or questioned my career choices, but I'd never thought of moving on from medicine, quitting, or giving up. And the Generational Health program really saved me during my period of burnout because it was a distractor and something that I could sink my energy into. As I watched my colleagues participate in the Generational Health program, and as I looked at what we had built together, I realized it was an antidote for them as well. It was a way for all of us to reappreciate our roles and responsibilities for the health and well-being of others. It was our sassafras, our careful dosing of medicine to dispel the burnout, reinstate our passion, and remind us of why we gave our lives to this calling.

This book is a compilation of stories from me, Kelly, and the dedicated caregivers and providers who have worked alongside us. Their stories memorialize their legacies of human connection.

—Diane Wintz (San Diego, California)

Part One

To practice medicine or nursing is to care for a stranger with dignity and compassion; to support the health-care journey with attention and caring; to provide comfort with knowledge and education; to bring solace in crisis and humility in miracles; to calm and allay fear, pain, or suffering; and to render treatment or interventions, acknowledging that the patient is the greatest expert of his or her own body and life.

Human Connection

To connect with others is the crux of human experience. In medicine, human connection is the magic sauce for successful hospitalization or discharge. It is needed for cohesive communication among team members, for a team approach to solving a mutual chronic problem, for treating an illness, or for recovering from surgery. It is the compassion behind the action; the soft place to fall when one is hurt; the support for the ill, injured, dying, or grieving; the most innate part of who we are, fulfilling that most basic need of life.

MANY PATIENTS TELL ME they feel the hospital is an extension of their home, where they feel comfortable and welcome. Some of my older patients were born in the same hospital where they now receive care. Their personal history includes the hospital. It is the location of miracles and of tragedies. We feel something when we walk through the door. The smell of a familiar hospital carries memories. The sensory data that we don't even realize brings us back to certain times in our memories when our lives were changed forever.

Despite all that, I find that people who are hospitalized don't actually want to be there. They don't mind visiting and going home, but when it comes to being a patient who cannot leave, that is when I see the frustration at the situation, anger at the disease, or disappointment in the team. I think clinicians play a vital role in how each patient views their own mortality or their own journey. Clinicians reflect the emotions, but it is critical for them to do it respectfully and to fully listen and be mindful of what matters to that person.

My job is to connect the patient with the care team and ensure they feel listened to and respected. I take the time to get to know someone and express gratitude for the opportunity to care for them. Yes, it is a job. But it is also my passion and my mission.

—Tracy, advanced illness nurse (Coronado Island, California)

In 2018, I was approached by a physician champion to consider a new role as coordinator of a program focusing on older, injured patients. I had been a nurse at the same ED for eight years, I had achieved a position in the trauma room, and I was not looking to do something different. In fact, I was baffled as to why anyone thought I would be interested. Trauma was so fast-paced, and that was my style and my training. I thrived on working with young people who had sustained massive injuries, resuscitating them, and then getting them to the ICU before repeating all the steps again for the next patient. Leadership wanted to take me out of that role, and I couldn't see the value at first.

There was a growing trend in the trauma population, though. The baby boomer generation was getting older, and they were living longer. I started to see more patients who were sixty-five and older than I ever had in the trauma room, and that wasn't going to revert. There was sustainability in geriatrics. I saw it everywhere, including with my parents. They were aging, and they were healthy, and they continued to do things that I always thought were "younger-people sports." If either of them was ever injured, I knew what they would fear most would be their loss of independence, and I wanted to impact that.

This position was going to be synonymous with a macroscopic move—one that would put me in front of administration regularly, give me a powerful voice, and enhance my career with the experience of building a program that hadn't existed previously. Since the program was new, and I was the coordinator, I would be responsible for showcasing the progress of the program's development. While there would be a medical director who would provide some ideas, the program would ultimately be mine to manage. I called my mom—who is also a nurse—and after talking it over with her, I really couldn't find a reason to say no. If it wasn't successful, I would just go back to my original position when the six-month pilot program was over. But I also had a chance to build something sustainable and lasting for our patients. And I found myself excited to get started.

One of the first things I did was to determine a mechanism to enroll patients into the program. I would meet with people who were being admitted to the trauma service, and I would talk to them about how life was at home. We would fill out a

FRAIL questionnaire[6] together, and then I would enroll them in a variety of therapy sessions during their hospitalization.

There was one patient who really stood out for me. He granted me the greatest compliment I could have received, which was that he didn't want to let me down. He knew the program was new and that it was a pilot. He knew I was a new coordinator. At one point, he said to his physical therapist, "I am really tired, and I don't want to get out of bed, but I don't want to let Jennifer down."

In that moment, I realized the type of difference I was making. That memory brings tears to my eyes. It was profound. This man, who was in his eighties and hurting, cared about how I felt, and he realized his participation (or lack of) might affect others. I'd really made a difference to him; he was working that hard on getting out of bed because he cared about how I felt. The human connection was the difference. The two of us sitting together and filling out a five-question template on his frailty was our bonding moment, and out of that came someone who changed our program forever.

I will never forget how that made me feel. It also fueled my fire because I wanted to be the solution. I wanted to show injured, older adults that they could participate in this program, and they could realistically get home again. I was tired of seeing fear and loss of independence, and through the program, I could make an impact.

In my twenty-five years of trauma bedside experience, this was the first opportunity for me to build bonds and relationships. This was the first time I could engage with patients, sit with them, and hear their stories. And it was life-changing for me. I really fell into this somewhat unwillingly, but when my six months were over, I craved the feeling that the program had given me.

And everyone was right. The coordinator role prepared me for the leadership position that came next, which was to manage the trauma program. Our trauma program encounters about 2,500 trauma patients per year, and one-third of them are over the age of sixty-four. It is significant, and I am so proud to have been involved in the initial growth and development.
—Jennifer, trauma program manager (San Diego, California)

Brian was on his bucket-list trip, riding cross-country on his motorcycle. His wife had had the foresight to put a tracker on the bike to set her mind at ease. About one hundred miles outside of San Diego, California, he swerved to avoid a deer, laid the motorcycle down, and wasn't able to call for help. The tracker was extremely helpful because it enabled emergency crews to find him and transport him to the hospital. His work-up revealed that he had a severe neck injury. The bones of his spine were disconnected from his skull. He had spinal injuries, a spinal cord injury, and bony fractures of his arms and legs. His risk of mortality from these injuries was high. His wife made the trip to town and supported the numerous surgeries he needed: spinal fusion, tracheostomy, and dozens of other operations to stabilize the injuries.

A couple of months later, he was ready to leave the hospital setting. He first went to a nursing facility and then came back to our hospital for formal rehabilitation. He made a complete, miraculous recovery.

Every year on the anniversary of his accident, he writes me a letter to remind me of his gratitude.

Dear doctor,

Two years ago today (May 2016), I was flown to the hospital in very bad condition after a serious motorcycle accident and was lucky enough to fall into your care. I had a cervical separation, broken neck, fractured leg, and broken ribs. I also had damage to my shoulder, both knees, an ankle, four cranial nerves, and various other parts on all corners of my body. While I was hospitalized, my family was told that I may not make it. If I did, they needed to be prepared for life-altering issues.

After all that, though, if you saw me today, you would not know that I had once been in the condition I was in. You, and the team you put together, did nothing short of a miraculous job.

Eight weeks after arriving, I was discharged home to Florida.

On this second anniversary, I would like to thank you again for all you did and provide you with an update.

I was admitted in May of 2016, as you know! I went back to Florida to a nursing care home in July, and by the end of the month, I quit all pain medications, muscle relaxants, and sleep aids. I didn't like how they made me feel. In August, I returned to abbreviated duty at work two days a week with my walker in tow. In October, I was approved for long-term disability, and shortly thereafter returned to full-time employment. Over the following few months I had at least five more surgeries. My paralyzed vocal cord and decreased hearing were related to cranial nerve damage and couldn't be fixed. I have virtually no pain in my neck. The left leg that sustained so much trauma has no issues at all.

This past spring, I walked in a five-kilometer race just to prove I could.

If you have the opportunity, please thank everyone who helped me. The care I received was amazing.

When meeting with a new doctor, the conversation is always the same. They ask about my injuries, I explain them, and they never believe me. Each time a doctor reads my medical history, they stare at me in shock and tell me I am a miracle. They can't believe I have recovered, returned to work, or live a normal life.

I've learned that people with my injuries don't survive. But I did. You and the team are the reason I live a very normal, happy, productive life.

Lastly, my wife asks that I pass along a hello for you. She simply states that you were my guardian angel.

If you ever find yourself in Florida, dinner is on us. There is so much we could tell you and bring you up to date.

Finally, if there is ever anything I can do to help any patient of yours or a patient you are aware of, let me know. It is likely I understand a bit of what they are going through, and if nothing else, I am an example of what can happen with medical care and some tenacity on their part.

Sincerely and with deepest thanks,
B

This past May of 2025 was Brian's ninth anniversary.

Nine years and still kicking. Thank you to you and all those you work with daily!

I retired at the end of the year. At sixty-four years old, it was my time. My wife and I are living a pleasantly normal life trying to find a new rhythm after so many years working. I had the most productive years of my career after I returned from bumping my head. Go figure that out …

My health has been good. Everything still works, and motorcycles are still banned. I had my physical with my primary care doctor this month. You got me fixed, and he keeps me up and running.

To you and all those you work with, thank you. I can't begin to count the number of people who cared for me. The ED team, the doctors and surgeons, nurses, occupational and physical therapists, neuropsychologists, technicians, radiologists, and on and on … all focused on me and put me back together again. Thank you.

I've mentioned this before, but it's stayed with me: An ICU nurse told me that his team rarely heard from patients after they left the hospital. They rarely saw recovery. If I had never been injured, I wouldn't have realized the weight of caring for someone who had been so critically injured, only to never know what happened to them. Let the ICU team know that even in the worst-case scenarios, patients fully recover because of them, because of their attention and care. I had a devastating injury and little hope, but I went on to have a full recovery and went back to living a fulfilling life with my beautiful wife, who I started dating when we were teens. That was the impact all those who work at the hospital had on me, whether they know it or not.

Thank you *everyone* for all you do every day. It makes a difference!

The fine print: For those who ask and may not know about the "bump on my head," you have my permission to tell them anything. I've made no secret of my accident, the journey, or the results. Feel free to discuss it as you wish.

PS: Here is a funny story. I went in for a routine colonoscopy. Someone from the practice called and wanted to know my medical history. I was already chuckling at the humor in my situation. She wanted to know every surgery I'd had. I tried to give her a way out and asked if she wanted just the major surgeries. She was unrelenting and wanted me to list them all. I listed all I could think of, and she dutifully typed them into my record. After I got off the phone, I remembered more.

Thanks for putting up with me, and thank you for being there nine years ago! There would be no me without you and your team.

With much respect and appreciation,
Brian, trauma survivor (Florida)

Some time ago, I cared for an older, homeless gentleman named Michael who had been run over and brought to the ED for evaluation. He was very appreciative of the care.

While I was explaining his injuries, which included many rib fractures, and was telling him about the plan to continue hospitalization, he said, "I'm a tough old bird, aren't I?"

And I agreed with him; he certainly was tolerating the pain well and had been through a traumatic event. He'd cared for himself on the street and managed all of his affairs without help or support. He was tough, without a doubt. But then, with tears in his eyes, he said, "I don't feel very tough right now."

I felt really deflated when he said that, and I wanted to give him something that would bring him back up, but there really wasn't anything I could do in that moment. He stayed in the hospital for two weeks before being placed in a facility for long-term recovery.

I thought often about Michael and how symbolic his story was. I'd focused on his care, on his well-being, and on acclimating him to a new injury in an older body that he was used to controlling. He was used to running the streets, he was respected there, and now he was an injured bird who needed a helping hand. It was the push and pull between what was right and best for his recovery, for his peace of mind, and for the service aspect of medicine versus the barriers dictated by his socioeconomic status and psychosocial factors. There was a vulnerability in being worn ragged by acquired helplessness, an inability to read, an inability to advocate for self, and a lack of knowledge on how to navigate the system. He needed a friend the most. He needed someone to listen to his needs and fears, and support him in these significant changes of life. He needed a doctor less. Sure, he needed medication management for pain. But what was he going to do with a recommendation for screening or instructions on using a medical portal to check his labs? He didn't have a phone. He was an unrepresented adult, now an older man, trying to figure out how he was going to survive institutionalization or how he would ever return to his home: the streets. His tent was fair game for anyone who realized he wasn't returning any time soon.

My connection with him made a difference. Not just for getting him placed over the long term and ensuring his safety, comfort, and health. But also for me and my understanding of the realities of life for so many people for whom health care is not accessible.

I heard later that he'd invested in his recovery process. He wanted to continue to live and write chapters. He adjusted to his life's circumstances. He wasn't done just because the world around him was changing. He learned to navigate his new circumstances with his own expertise. Being contemporary, challenged, and intelligent—or tough—was important to his identity.

I smiled. It wasn't just him walking away with something of value. I knew that my connection to him had created that opportunity, and I allowed myself to be proud of what I had been able to do for him: to support him, to validate his importance in his own life and in mine, and to look at this man who was so different from me, so rough around the edges, and see a life that had meaning.

—Diane Wintz (San Diego, California)

Compassion, Dignity, and Free Will

In every health-care journey is a person with a life story, family, friends, aspirations, expectations, and hope for the future. Life colors each individual's experience, influencing how a patient internalizes information about their health or makes decisions. Just as judgment in medicine is reserved for providing options and supporting patients through informed decision-making, rather than for opinions or assumptions to rationalize disease or one's state of health, so, too, do health-care experts enable and empower compassion in their care; dignity to the sick, ill, or injured; and free will to their patients.

JOSEPH HAD FALLEN FROM a great height while working on his ranch. He'd sustained a neck injury that rendered him paralyzed, quadriplegic, and unable to move anything below his shoulders. He couldn't feed himself or provide any of his self-care. Breathing was difficult. Very soon, he was exhausted by it and required permanent placement of a tracheostomy and support from a ventilator. He mouthed words and continued to make his own decisions. He was completely awake and aware of the world around him.

His family was incredibly supportive and positive, but it eventually became apparent that he was living for *their* happiness, not his own. When they left the hospital for the night, he would suddenly refuse all interventions and tell his nurses (soundlessly, mouthing words) that he wanted to be done.

The nursing team brought their concerns forward. Was he just agreeing to interventions because he thought his family expected that? The medical team reapproached him and asked him directly if he was living solely because that was his family's expectation?

He nodded and then explained that he had too much anxiety about them. How would they go on without him? What about the finances of the ranch? What about the cost of his care going forward? How could he never go home again and agree to live in a nursing facility for the rest of his life? They couldn't take care of him, and he didn't want them to. He didn't want them to feel obligated to care for him—full-time, helping with everything—and essentially give their time and their lives to him when he wasn't really living anymore. This wasn't the quality of life that he wanted. Living like this was akin to a prison sentence from which he could never escape. He wasn't going to be able to enjoy family events. He was going to be stuck on a ventilator in a nursing home while living and waiting for someone to visit; and for him, that was torture. He had been active and had lived on a working ranch his entire life, seventy years. He could not adjust and didn't want to adjust to a life with minimal activity and interactions that were only to support his health or his hygiene. This wasn't depression or an adjustment to disease. This was a new, unfamiliar life, and he didn't want it.

His family arrived later that day to visit, and the medical team met with them outside the room. They were shocked and disappointed that they could be sending the wrong message. They wanted him to be happy, and if that meant stopping the life support, then they would back him up in converting his care to a comfort-focused plan where a natural death could occur. It was ultimately his decision, and they wanted him to know they were OK with it.

I watched outside the room as they went in and hugged him. He couldn't hug them back because he had no ability to move or lift his arms. Everyone was teary-eyed as the ventilator was disconnected, and he drifted slowly to sleep and then peacefully passed away. It was his will and his choice to no longer pursue the care plan. It also would have been acceptable to continue the machine-driven support, but it wasn't what he wanted. It felt good that he was able to be the master of his own medical plan, that he was trusted and capable of making his own decisions, and that he had the support from his family to do that.

—Anonymous, physician (Houston, Texas)

Ann was eighty-four years old and lived alone. Prior to the COVID-19 pandemic, she had actively engaged in her local community center, learned different types of dances, exercised, and learned about her basic health maintenance from nursing students who volunteered there. Her faith was very important to her, and it manifested through her time spent at church and making rosaries for her community. This was her social life: spending time with a group of other church members, all talking, sharing about their families, and planning events. Ann also volunteered to visit those who were unable to drive to the church. She liked to provide home visits to the older adults who could no longer join the congregation in person. One of them taught her how to play cards, which brought moments of togetherness, well-being, and connectedness. Practicing her faith and being of service to others were meaningful parts of her life. Then, due to the pandemic, the community center closed and attending church services became a health risk.

Ann shared that her loneliness during COVID-19 was overwhelming due to the social isolation. She frequently called her friends to stay in touch, but her sense of community and connectedness were blunted with not being in person anymore. The community center was slow to reopen following the height of the pandemic, and she fell, rendering her hospitalized. Her increased sense of loneliness and isolation was a story familiar to many older adults.

Promotion of patient-centered care was one of my priorities. As a chaplain, I assessed how people made meaning out of life by understanding their anchored values and beliefs. I prioritized reconnecting to those anchors during times of struggle or illness, including with the help of spiritual or religious practices that nurtured the soul.

Loneliness and isolation are recognized as key social determinants of geriatric health, and they were most notable during the pandemic when there was a worldwide shutdown of social outlets. Age also brings changes in hearing or ability to effectively communicate. Adult children grow up and leave the nest to start their own families, and there is a consistent drive to not be a "burden."

In a hospital setting, this loneliness can present as a lack of support for making decisions or insufficient help after discharge, the thought of which can cause extra anxiety, fear of illness or injury, or conversely, using the hospital as a social refuge. In my role as chaplain and manager of volunteer services, I seek to recognize these issues early on so that I can offer resources to fill the gaps and provide the necessary support. Volunteers offer activities related to arts and crafts and music. Some help our patients tell their stories and create posters so that visitors and staff coming into their rooms can learn about the patients. Energy modalities like healing touch and Reiki, comfort hand massage, and pet therapy are effective ways to reduce stress and nurture joy. These extras emphasize what is important to the person receiving them.

Supporting aging adults requires a team effort that includes other disciplines such as social workers and case managers who work together with each patient for a safe discharge. The discharge planning takes into consideration the patient's medical needs and the environment that will best support their recovery and well-being. I often see this mutual sense of gratitude emerging through this multiservice effort that soothes that sense of loneliness and serves to rekindle one's ability to connect with others. This is the power of being seen and feeling heard.

During Ann's hospitalization, she received visits from various volunteers and chaplains. These interactions served her need to feel appreciated and appreciate others, to understand her value, and to reconnect with her spiritual practice and faith. Our team was also a beneficiary of her wisdom. After a time, she was able to go home and to live independently with the help of a caregiver. Not all our patient encounters have such endings, but we are called to listen and to respond in a manner that we hope is contributing to the welfare of our patients and our community.

—Mica, manager for spiritual care, volunteers, and education (San Diego, California)

My dad was the kind of guy whose gruff exterior often spoke louder than his words, his no-nonsense attitude a constant reminder that life was about getting things done, not talking about them. In contrast, my mom was the quiet force behind the scenes, a woman of few words and an unspoken sense of strength. Her awkwardness in certain situations was covered up by an infectious giggle that made anyone who met her smile. Together, they made an unlikely yet perfect pair, balancing each other in ways we never fully understood but always admired.

In 2016, my dad was diagnosed with terminal stomach cancer. I flew back to Bhutan to assist with his treatment options. We got first, second, and third opinions from physicians and specialists—and all of them had the same consensus.

The tumor was inoperable since my dad was physically too frail at the time of diagnosis to undergo surgery. The recommendation was chemotherapy and radiation. After many discussions, my dad decided he did not want further treatment. My dad lived for seven months after this diagnosis. While palliative care services were not available in Bhutan at this time, his symptoms and pain were effectively managed. He passed away peacefully in the home he and my mom had built, where they'd raised the four of us. I believe his last seven months were a gift because he got to spend time with people who mattered to him, to say his goodbyes, and to live life on his terms without much pain or suffering. For my mom, his peaceful passing provided some solace.

After my dad passed away, I kept hearing about people I knew who had passed away from cancer. Some of these stories highlighted the patient's pain and suffering while alive. In death, they left their families with regret and trauma. Hearing these stories showed me the need for palliative and end-of-life services in Bhutan. It was then that I decided to go back to school for my doctoral degree to learn about program implementation and evidence-based project development and to enhance my own knowledge of these valuable services.

I was in my last year of school when my mom was diagnosed with stage four lung cancer. Once again, I made the journey home to assist with her care and treatment. Having previously survived cervical cancer, my mom tolerated the several rounds of chemotherapy and radiation exceptionally well. However, a few months later, she was admitted to the hospital for respiratory issues. This time, I was surprised to learn that a fledgling palliative care program had been introduced in Bhutan. The program had four nurses who worked closely with a medical oncologist. However, the program was only based in the capital city of Thimphu and served patients who were referred from the local hospital. The nurses themselves had no palliative experience or training. Palliative visits to my mom were often limited to asking how she was doing. There were no assessments and no discussions about care goals or interventions for symptom management.

After my mom had been in the hospital for several months, the oncologist suggested discontinuing chemotherapy since it was no longer proving to be beneficial. Despite this change in her treatment plan, my mom seemed to be doing well. She was close to being discharged, and I was preparing to return to America when her condition suddenly deteriorated. My mom's lungs and heart were starting to give out. As the care team tried various interventions, the last words I heard my mom whisper were, "Enough. I'm so tired."

The doctors provided us with two options: intubation and admission to the ICU, or comfort care. The medical consensus was that her prognosis was poor and that her chance of recovery in the ICU was minimal. Knowing that an ICU admission would mean she would be sedated and alone during what could be her final hours, the family made the difficult decision to accept comfort care. She could spend her last moments in her private room surrounded by her children, family, and many grandchildren.

While we understood the impending loss, I was grateful for this last time with her. She was no longer conscious, but we were able to connect her with her siblings around the world. They talked to her on the phone, prayed with and for her, and said their final goodbyes. And as she started to decline further, I told her we would be OK and that she could let go to reunite with Dad. Eventually, in the early hours of that morning, her heart stopped, and she passed away peacefully surrounded by family. As I turned off the cardiac monitors and called the nurses to let them know of her passing, I found consolation in the fact that her last moments had been filled with the voices and presence of those she loved and those who loved her. Each of my parents were seventy-six years old at the time of their passing.

Meanwhile, on the other side of town, unbeknownst to me, one of my best friends was going through the same situation.

However, hers was a traumatic experience as she watched her mother suffer until the end. When I visited her shortly after my mom's passing to offer my condolences, my friend's trauma and grief were heartbreaking. Her experience stayed with me as I returned to America. It made me more determined to assist in any way I could to improve palliative and end-of-life care services in Bhutan.

Back in America, I was assigned a position on the surgical arm of Generational Health. I was coordinating education for surgical vulnerabilities and working with nursing from the Advanced Illness Management team to ensure open communication between patients and their care teams. AIM nurses were instrumental in supporting patients through the transition to palliative care when surgical options were exhausted. As I explored ways to assist palliative care services in Bhutan, I found a volunteer organization called Health Volunteers Overseas (HVO).[7] HVO had an oncology project in Bhutan and was also providing patient consultations to the four nurses in the new palliative care program.

As an advanced practice clinical nurse specialist (APRN-CNS), my area of expertise is in nursing education, program development, and project implementation. And as a Bhutanese, I felt my cultural knowledge would be helpful to liaison between the Bhutan and HVO teams. I joined the HVO-Bhutan project in 2020. At that time, on-site visits to Bhutan had been discontinued due to the pandemic, and virtual education sessions on Wednesday nights (morning in Bhutan) were in progress. During these sessions, an HVO volunteer would virtually review complex palliative care cases with the nurses or provide didactic education on pharmacology, pathophysiology of chronic and oncology-related diseases, nursing assessments, nursing diagnoses, and symptom management. Soon after, I was asked to take over as the co-country director for the palliative care project.

Today, the palliative program continues to grow. The focus now is no longer on nursing education as the Bhutanese nurses feel confident in their practice. Instead, the program has transitioned to peer-to-peer palliative care training for nurses at hospitals around Bhutan. These training sessions ensure that this valuable service will also be accessible to patients at the community level throughout the country.

Last year, I made my first visit to Bhutan since my mom's passing. I was fortunate enough to meet with health leadership and share my passion for palliative care and the HVO mission. Earlier this year, through a fully funded HVO scholarship, two Bhutanese nurses had the opportunity to spend two weeks in Singapore to observe and learn about best practices in palliative and hospice care. Since their return, they have been working on improving nursing assessments, patient referral systems, and program enhancement. More recently, I was honored to be part of the team that aided the nurses in creating a project proposal for Bhutan's first hospice service to be implemented in the latter part of 2025.

As I look back on my personal journey with palliative and end-of-life care services in Bhutan, I am inspired by the commitment and compassion of the Bhutanese nurses who, despite having meager resources, strive to provide the best possible care to their vulnerable patients. I am humbled and thankful to my HVO volunteer colleagues who have given and continue to give so generously of their time, expertise, and resources. There is no doubt that I still have a long road ahead before I realize my personal goal of having these services available in every health-care facility in Bhutan, and to every Bhutanese family who needs it, but I am so excited and grateful that our journey has begun!

—Thuji, clinical nurse specialist (Bhutan)

My husband, Terry, was eighty-five years young when he tripped over the garden hose in the backyard. He felt an immediate sting in his hands and pain in his neck. I called 911, unsure of what would happen next. At the hospital, we were told he had a severe neck injury and would need surgery.

Over the next few days, as his surgeons prepared for the operation, Terry and I had many conversations about life.

Terry loved gardening and being outside. He cherished being home with me, and he enjoyed a home-cooked meal, a glass of red wine, and good conversation. We had been each other's world since high school, always making decisions together. Now he faced a surgery with uncertain outcomes regarding recovery, independence, and returning home.

I had been diagnosed with breast cancer a few years ago, and now it was advanced. I wasn't sure how much time I had left, and I worried about what would happen to Terry when I was gone. Who would help him with his recovery? There seemed to be short-term solutions, but nothing for the long term.

Terry consented to the surgery because the alternative was unthinkable: living with a neck injury and constant fear of paralysis.

The surgery went smoothly, but the recovery was challenging.

Terry was in constant pain and needed medication all the time. This weighed heavily on him. He didn't want to move because of the pain, and he often couldn't feel his hands and described them as being "asleep." He needed help with everything, even brushing his teeth. The biggest issue was that he couldn't swallow. He choked on everything, even his own saliva. Despite following all the medical advice, he wasn't improving.

About two weeks after the operation, he was offered a feeding tube. He listened politely as the doctor explained it, but when the doctor left, Terry looked at me and said, "I don't want to do this anymore."

We were unsure of our options. Was a feeding tube necessary? Could we refuse it? What would happen if we did? Would he feel like he was starving? Generational Health supported us through the process and spent time with us at his bedside so that we could understand the options.

What happened next was heartbreaking. Terry was moved to hospice after refusing the feeding tube. The Generational Health team explained that, without the ability to eat or sustain nutrition and hydration, he would die naturally. The focus then shifted to treating his discomfort.

Terry's death was both the worst and best day of my life. It was the worst because I lost my best friend, partner, and beloved husband of more than sixty years. It was the best because I knew he was no longer miserable. Accepting comfort care and hospice was the right choice for both of us. I don't carry the burden of wondering what would have happened to him when I go or feeling like I contributed to his pain.

—Janice, Terry's wife (Houston, Texas)

Inescapable Truths

Disease, illness, and injury are inescapable during the course of natural life. Despite the innate knowledge that health declines and is not something to take for granted, when a health event happens, it is often a surprise, rearing when least expected, when one is on a smooth path of life and not seeking problems. The unpredictability of health drives fear, anger, frustration, and appreciation for wellness, a craving for the health issue to move from center stage. The state of health changes the perspective of life's journey, and priorities shift to accommodate the new normal with a constant need for empathy, meaning, or the why as an explanation.

WHEN I WAS ON my first rotation as an intern, I took care of an eleven-year-old with congenital liver failure. She was listed for transplant with the expectation that hospitalization would continue until a transplant was available or until her body gave out, whichever came first.

Every day, I would visit her and her mother who were waiting and wondering if any news would come. Day after day, they waited on a donor, on a match, on news. Every day, they wondered if they would hear something. I found myself holding my breath for them each time I knocked on the door to go in and say hello. I thought about what an eleven-year-old girl's life was supposed to be like: summer camp, sports, friends, maybe a first crush, body changes, and so much promise and excitement for what the future held. And then I would go into the room and see an eleven-year-old who was jaundiced, sick, and felt terrible with liver-induced confusion and lethargy. It wasn't fair. It wasn't the way it was supposed to be.

And then, one day while I was in the room, the phone rang, and the voice on the other end of the line said that there was a liver available. After weeks of waiting and wondering and knowing that a match may not occur, the transplant coordinator had given the lifesaving news that this little girl was going to get a liver. And prior to that phone call, there had been the twenty-one-year-old who had been involved in a fatal car accident, rendering a liver available to a matching recipient.

I wanted to jump up and down, scream, and cry because that moment was one of the best of my life. I held my breath for weeks while we provided critical care and organ support. I knew how risky the surgery was going to be, but I wanted to celebrate that one moment when everything felt like it was going to be OK, and I could breathe again. I could go home and not think about this mom and her anxiety and her prayer for her daughter. I could feel good about not thinking about her.

I heard the whir of the helicopter's propeller. My heart was beating loudly in my chest. The emotions twisted and turned between thoughts of one mom who was hopeful and terrified and another mom who was mourning the death of her son. One child would live because another child had died. How can you celebrate and be in mourning at the same time? There was a transplant match after waiting for weeks. There was one compatible liver in the nation for one person who wouldn't survive without it.

I could feel my heart beating in my chest as the helicopter landed with the liver inside. The liver was delivered on a machine that continued its perfusion until it could be safely transplanted. The girl was brought to the operating room, and the surgery started in an effort to save her life, the only chance to save her.

We didn't have a way to know that she wouldn't make it. We didn't have a way to stop the massive hemorrhage that occurred. We didn't have a way to transfuse her quickly enough. After the somber walk to the conference room with the transplant surgeon, I sat down face to face with her mother. The "I'm sorry" was the last thing I heard. "I'm sorry," and life would never be the same. It felt like all the air had been sucked out of the room. All the hope and anticipation was gone. It was dark, dark, dark … there was no sound but the sigh of defeat. Failure overwhelmed the space.

—Anonymous (San Diego, California)

Jason and I had been married for forty-eight hours, and it was finally time for our honeymoon in Costa Rica. Jungles, beaches, and other outdoor adventures.

On day one, we landed and embarked on the scenic drive to our treehouse-style accommodations. We were greeted with fresh passion fruit juice and enjoyed an authentic dinner under the stars.

On day two, we ventured out to zipline, received more tropical fruit along the way, and got our bearings.

On day three, we went hiking.

On day four, we woke up to a voicemail: "Jason, this is the oncologist regarding your blood work. Please give us a call back as soon as possible."

"Oncologist?"

Jason hadn't been sick. He didn't have any health problems. In fact, he'd had a routine physical about a month before we had gotten married. We had planned to combine our insurance plans, so in order for him to switch over, he had to do a complete exam and lab work. Was this some sort of mistake call?

While pacing the hotel room, unable to get any phone calls to connect to the outside world, we managed to reach my sister by text. She is a physician and tried to give us some peace of mind. She reminded us that he was overall healthy. However, we were rattled during the rest of the trip and were unable to get resolution until we returned home.

Upon retesting his blood levels, we were in and out of doctors' offices, with the final consensus being that his white blood cell count was above normal, which led to a diagnosis of chronic lymphocytic leukemia (CLL).[8]

A cancer diagnosis.

Racing through my mind were the thoughts that I didn't want him to be sick and I didn't know what this meant for our life together. We wanted to grow a family, but could we?

I was so excited to have found him and to be married, and it felt like we were hit with a catastrophe right off the bat. Here we were in this milestone moment of getting married, being on a honeymoon, and planning a family, and we were facing a cancer diagnosis that was brand-new and terrifying.

How had we found ourselves here? My stomach fell to my knees.

The first few months of this new nomenclature were a whirlwind. Doctors' visits, a scary liver biopsy, second and third opinions, and deciding which treatment would be best. In early 2018, some doctors were still promoting a low-dose form of chemotherapy while others were touting stem cell clinical trials. We didn't understand why there were so many different opinions for the same disease. If you have pneumonia, you get antibiotics. No one expects you to choose your medical therapy with a disease. But Jason's cancer was a completely different experience. We were expected to choose the therapy and treatment plan based on a variety of options offered while understanding only a fraction of the lingo.

Today, after a three-year regimen of immunotherapy, Jason has been off the medication and rarely gets sick. While it's likely that his white blood cell count will spike again, we are thankful for our best-case, long-term scenario with a cancer diagnosis.

Due to the urgency in those first few months, we quickly realized our plan to wait a year before family planning would be impossible. I had envisioned us traveling more and enjoying our new marriage before having children. We knew we wanted at least one child, and the window to get pregnant was extremely small given everything we were dealing with. In 2018, there was no data on CLL patients as young as Jason. The medication was strong with unknown side effects to a potential fetus. And so began our dive into the world of in vitro fertilization (IVF) to buy us more time and an "insurance policy" for having our own family.

Suddenly, it was sperm banks, needles, storage fees, covert shots in public bathrooms, more doctor shopping, financial aid, hormones, doubt, fear, failure—and finally, success. We know how lucky we are that it only took one IVF attempt to get our incredible son, Reid.

My pregnancy was relatively uneventful, but unfortunately, I suffered a complicated and traumatic birth. This was the first time I had ever been hospitalized. I had never broken a bone. I was squeamish with gory movies, and I always cried during shots.

The situation in the delivery room escalated quickly. Jason was pacing around, nervous, and feeling the anxious energy from everyone. There was high blood pressure, widespread infection, meconium aspiration, hiccups with communication, and a heightening concern for me as I spiked a temperature of 106°F. It earned me an ICU stay and a short neonatal intensive care unit (NICU) residency for Reid.

I can't recall many of the events and details of my delivery and what followed. I was completely delirious with that high temperature. New parents always experience a mix of adrenaline and exhaustion in the first few days after a baby is born, but this was intensified. Jason was barely hanging on, and I had been hospitalized and had to recover for ten days. Again, though, we found our path and our way through. Today, our son Reid is a healthy, energetic five-year-old with no residual health concerns.

While we feel we have had enough medical scares and drama to last ten lifetimes, we learned and we grew together.

We realized how critical it was to rely on others and to stay positive. We didn't need to worry about every unknown or every possibility. We didn't have to spend our time together laser-focused on the things we could not control. We could—and did—choose to continue living and moving forward. We enjoyed inner-tube rides and hiking on our honeymoon. We had great dinners with many laughs, even during chemotherapy. We appreciated the process of fertility and got excited about how we would tell the family when I got pregnant. So much about those memories was amazing and great. But at the same time, it was eye-opening how life could change in a blink. What we thought we would plan and have control over was just a fantasy. Life goes the way it does; it will throw unexpected things your way, and it will be yours to discover the path through it.

—Helene, speech pathologist (Los Angeles, California)

Sometimes it is hard to acknowledge that even in an emergency, surgery is a choice that should only be made once all the risks and potential benefits are understood. In 2022, our team met with a patient who was in his eighties. He had a young son, and he wanted to see him graduate high school, but he needed an open-heart surgery. There were concerns about his surgical fitness and his ability to tolerate surgery based on his underlying functional status, which was poor. He was nutritionally depleted, and he wasn't walking much due to heart disease. We counseled him extensively about all the what-ifs, knowing that he would very likely have a complication (the question being which one). We reviewed every limitation that he had for himself regarding machine-driven support, and we established a chain of decision-makers. We were worried about him not being able to come off a ventilator when we would be offering another operation to place a tracheostomy (airway support) into his neck. We worried that his kidneys could fail, and that he might need dialysis. Would he want that? What if he had a stroke during or after the operation? That was a risk. Who would speak for him if he could not talk? What if he didn't make it through the surgery?

He would not survive without the operation, so he decided to go forward, fully informed about the risks. In the end, he did not have a single complication. Maybe we were so prepared that we provided everything he needed, including extensive support and education.

Preoperative counseling is one of my favorite parts of caring for people. We build a real connection by talking about the things that matter most and trying to meet goals together. From a provider's perspective, it feels great to provide a surgical solution and have a great outcome, restoring someone to the life they had before.

—Anonymous, cardiac surgeon (San Diego, California)

Residency was five long years of learning, practicing, and fielding darts poisoned with poignant insults and microaggressions meant to toughen me for a future career where self-confidence, judgment, and empathy needed to emerge from my polite, quiet, and scared inner child to give patients the best experience. My former mentor used to say, "Sometimes wrong, never in doubt." That pretty much summed up the cockiness needed to walk into a room and tell an adult stranger that they needed to trust me to operate on them.

As I grew into the career and went from being a novice, nervous resident to an experienced, expert surgeon, I realized there were pieces missing from my mentor's comment: the power of the past, the lessons learned, and intuition. The saying should have been, "Sometimes wrong, but willing to give my time to any complication or question, completely prepared having seen and experienced this before, caring about this person going through this experience, and trusting me to be their guide."

It was my last month as a surgical resident, and I was looking forward to fellowship where I would concentrate on critical care. Mrs. Miller was rolling into the OR to undergo a Whipple[9] operation (removal of the head of the pancreas and rerouting of the biliary structures) for her pancreatic cancer. She was anticipating a rough road. She had been counseled by her surgeon that even though he thought he could remove the cancer, she would still need adjuvant chemotherapy and possibly radiation. She felt sick all the time, though: nauseated and full. Her weight loss had been substantial, and her clothes were way too loose (and not in the way she always wanted to be skinny).

Her husband was rubbing her shoulders and hyping her up while she signed the consent form and listened to all the risks of the operation one last time. The surgical nurse verified that she was agreeable to surgery, placed an armband, covered her hair with a net, and reviewed the potential side effects of receiving a blood transfusion. Despite all of her nervous energy, she was excited for the surgery. It was her chance to get back to a normal life.

She closed her eyes as the anesthesiologist placed the oxygen mask on her face and told her to take deep breaths. She continued her silent, repetitive prayer: "Please, God, help me through this and help me get better." She started to count backward from one hundred but didn't make it to ninety-six before she was asleep. Her abdomen was prepped for surgery, and her surgeon (with me as the assistant) commenced her operation.

The cancer was more advanced than we'd thought, but we were still able to do a successful resection and complete the operation.

She woke up and went on to a recovery period of several weeks. I was able to visit her on the day of her discharge. I hopped into her room and saw that all her bags had been packed, she was dressed, and her IV had been removed.

But something was very wrong. Her color.

She was as white as a sheet. She had beads of sweat on her forehead. I knew within seconds of looking at her that she looked like death. I ran over to her bed and grabbed her hand. "Mrs. Miller, what is going on?"

Her eyes rolled back in her head. I pulled the Code Blue cord. People started running into the room, and it became very chaotic. They placed a new IV, swiftly placed a breathing tube to protect her airway, ran labs, put her back into a hospital gown, and rapidly transported her to the ICU with her husband trailing behind, lost and confused about what was going on.

Lab work showed she was bleeding. I called the operating room. She needed emergent surgery. Blood was transfusing as fast as possible as I alerted her husband of the plan and my concerns for her. I was scared she was going to die. In a trance, he signed the consent for her, and she was rolled back to the OR; this time, it was a rushed and hushed experience with everyone understanding the catastrophe before them.

I opened her abdomen as quickly as I could. Six liters of bright-red blood ran like a volcano. I packed, packed, and packed trying to get enough pressure from the bandages so that maybe it would slow down enough for me to find the source. I never did identify exactly what was hemorrhaging, but I assumed it was the tumor that had eroded into an artery. There was no way to save her. I knew that. I did everything I could, everything I knew to do, and her husband knew that.

He knew what I was going to say when he saw me walking toward him in the waiting room. He saw my shoe covers splattered with blood, he saw my fatigue and disappointment, he saw me deflated, and he knew. And he accepted it. And he thanked me for doing everything I could. We never saw each other again.

I called my mom on my way home that night. Sobbing, I told her what had happened. She sighed and reminded me that this event had happened in a hospital where there were experts who had experience. That level of decision-making and that alacrity of response were only possible within the hospital's walls. If this event had happened the next day, she would have been at home, and her husband would have been alone trying to save her. He would have carried that guilt and that emotion forever. The team had been her guardian angels and his, saving him from having that weight on his shoulders. We were experts who were equipped to deal with this level of emergency and catastrophe, better prepared to handle the medical issues and the emotions than he was, and we saved him that.

—Anonymous, general surgeon (Baltimore, Maryland)

Part Two

The practice of medicine is a unique calling that requires complete selfless devotion to patients in the worst moments of their lives, in the middle of the night, on holidays, and on weekends. There are no days off, and at any moment, someone could have an emergency that needs directed and immediate attention from the team. To give of yourself in this way, to give your time whenever needed, is unlike any other profession, and those who decide to pursue this career realize that it is a lifestyle, it is a responsibility, and it is an honor to care for people.

THE HARDEST QUESTION I ever had to answer was "Why do you want to be a doctor?" I wasn't sure how to convey my drive or motivation to get through training and later matriculate into this career of surgery. It was an obvious question to ask, but the answer was not straightforward, especially in an evolving health-care milieu and as my life and my priorities changed over time. Mentorship played a critical role for me, guiding me to a career in medicine—specifically surgery with a strong focus on trauma. I witnessed surgeon heroes perform miraculous surgeries on hemorrhaging and critically injured patients. I wanted to be in that world where I could impact the lives of others.

—Diane Wintz (San Diego, California)

What Matters Matters

The medical field is a profession that impacts people. Every medical action has a reaction that affects somebody's life and can impact their ability to return to independence or spend meaningful time with their family or their friends, or it can interfere with their ability to work or play. We shouldn't offer medical interventions without understanding what is important to our patients, how our interventions will affect them, the alternatives to treatment, or the options that would work better to get that person back to the life they want to live.

WHEN I ENCOUNTER PATIENTS in the hospital, it is rare to know much about that person. I typically do not find out about their life, their hobbies, or their career. I may only meet their family if they live locally and come to visit. The "what matters" issue is often a guess, as the thing in front of me, the problem I need to solve, is the medical illness or injury. Yet that is the crux of the issue. Medical teams have gotten away from getting to know the things that matter to their patients.

James "Red" Duke was an attending surgeon when I was a second-year resident on trauma. He had been on his call shift in Dallas, Texas, when President Kennedy was assassinated, and he was a hero to me and hundreds of thousands of patients, trainees, and students.

He and I were rounding on the inpatient service of seventy patients. The service was insanely busy with each patient having upward of ten listed injuries or issues. We walked from room to room, and he introduced himself, shook hands, sat down on the visitor bench, and posed personal questions to each patient like we were out to lunch. He was fully engaged in each person's story.

In one room, he joined a man to watch an old Western movie with John Wayne, and he told me to continue on without him. I couldn't believe it. Here I was running around like a headless chicken, trying to coordinate operations, consultants, and medications while also having critical conversations, keeping up with the lists of injuries, making phone calls, and examining every patient. And he had time to watch a movie. At what point would that happen for me? Would I ever get to relax in that way? Would I ever enjoy my time with patients?

I couldn't see it, but later in my career, this finally happened. I was able to slow down long enough to find out what mattered to people. What they really wanted out of their hospitalization. I was able to find my joy in caring for people, to learn about them, and to savor moments of their lives that mattered to them. And that was the point when my surgical career became a love instead of a duty.

—Diane Wintz (San Diego, California)

I met with Emma to talk to her about her upcoming surgery. Emma was eighty-four and still working full-time when she'd been in a car accident. She'd walked away from the accident with a little strain on her neck. Her primary care doctor had recommended physical therapy, which she'd attended religiously for three months. Unfortunately, her neck continued to cause chronic pain, and she started to think something was wrong.

She decided to go to the ED with her husband in tow. Once there, the medical team informed her that the injury had significantly progressed, and she now had an unstable cervical spine that was at risk of collapse and quadriplegia. She was advised that she needed emergency surgery.

The neurosurgeon was planning operative intervention that same day. She was full of energy, a pistol!

She told me, "Get on with it. I understand I could die, but this neck pain is unbearable. I've been like this for three months, and if this is it, then fine. But try the surgery, and let's see."

Her husband, Sam, who was present during the conversation, added, "I want the same thing. If I ever need surgery, and I'm not going to be OK afterward, just let me go. We are in agreement and have had a lot of talks about this."

And so she proceeded to have the surgery. When it came time to wake her up from anesthesia and remove her breathing tube to start her recovery process, we realized she'd had a major stroke. It was on the dominant side of her brain, and in the best-case scenario she would have been dependent on nursing care forever. I went to meet with Sam to give comfort.

We sat down in a conference room with no windows. There was nowhere to look but directly at him. I told him that Emma had had a stroke after her surgery. He swallowed. I watched him internalize the information, his face changing from hopeful to shocked to crestfallen to devastated to resigned. He heaved a heavy sigh. He uttered no words yet spoke volumes.

The stroke was not disappointing; it was catastrophic. It was a death sentence for Emma, who was eighty-four years old and had no interest in spending any time in a long-term care facility or being dependent on full-time care. Sam knew it, and so did I. I was so incredibly sad to be sitting in front of him, dejected and sick. I wanted to fix it, but I couldn't. I couldn't do anything. The damage had been done, and now we had to jump to next steps. We couldn't sit in the conference room all night. How long was enough time to receive this information, accept it, and make the decisions that needed to be made?

I told him he didn't have to do anything that night. We could wait until morning and reevaluate everything with fresh eyes. He put his warm hand on mine.

He looked right at me, sighed again, and puffed. "I know exactly what she would want me to do. I don't need to wait until morning. I can hear her yelling at me now. 'Sam, you know what the hell I want. Just do it already.' We had so many conversations about what was important to us, how we wanted to get older, what we needed life to look like. Oh my God, I am not ready to let her go, but I know that I have to."

And then he burst into sobs, let go of my hand, and put his head on the table while he gasped. "I know what she wants."

I waited for him to walk back to her ICU room.

Emma's nurse gave me the look that said it all. Sam nodded. Medications were hung, and he grabbed Emma's hand and sat in the metal chair that had been waiting for him. He told her it was OK to go, and then he went through the story of their first date. Emma's heart rate slowed until there was no more rhythm seen on the heart monitor.

Sam left the hospital several hours later, holding a bag of her belongings. He looked lost. But right before he walked through the doors to leave the ICU, he turned around, and I saw him say, "I knew what she wanted. I knew what mattered. I knew what was important."

—Anonymous, Generational Health nurse (San Diego, California)

As a chaplain, I'm a spiritual care provider. I spend my time between the NICU and the adult ICUs, and as such, I get to see the bookends of life, the very beginning and the end. I have often thought about the similarities of care needs in these two extremes of life.

A baby or a neonate is dependent upon caregivers or dependent upon healers for every basic need. As a baby becomes a child and grows into their teenage years, there is a struggle for independence, to cruise down the highway in a car purchased from earnings in a first job, to break curfew, to enter higher-level education or a career, to start a family and create a home and memories. Then there comes a point in time when an adult becomes dependent again on others for basic living, and their grown child may move into a parenting role. The adult child is now responsible for confiscating the car keys from their parent. The older adult is no longer able to live in the family residence and now needs constant supervision or nursing care. That arc of life swings at those extremes of age where we must rely upon each other at the beginning and at the end of life.

One of the other things that I notice is physical frailty. A baby—very tender, very fragile—needs to be treated with care. They haven't yet learned about danger, and they don't know how to survive without support. The same level of fragility comes with age. Dementia may take the rationale and reasonability of life, or there may be physical changes, weakness, or instability with movement. Growing older may warrant a new level of tender loving care and attention, more help than before, and acceptance for the changes that are happening. And again, the arc of life goes full circle.

A baby learns about the world in the way that their consciousness can. Each experience is new and emotional with an opportunity to learn a life lesson. An adult has lived decades in a body that they have grown to know, but with age must learn to adapt to change. Just like a baby learns to adjust to their surroundings, an older adult acclimates to this body that may no longer feel familiar.

I notice the importance of social and human connection. In the neonatal ICU, kangaroo care is encouraged.[10] The baby is held skin to skin with the adult for bonding. It is wonderful for the baby. It is how the baby feels nurtured and loved. That touch and warmth provide the basic needs of comfort and love. When I go to the bedside of someone who is in the later years of life, I often realize the power of human touch, the need to not be alone, and the craving for human connection.

I notice the benefit of intergenerational bonding with parents and grandparents or other family members in the perinatal and neonatal worlds. Generations of people take care of and love a little baby, providing support and nurturing, maturing to the provision of life lessons as the child grows. We need that same support as we grow older. We need people who are around our age and younger than us, and potentially even older than us. We need those bonds.

The other things that strike me in terms of the parallels are the chapters of life. For any baby, there is a story still to be written. Everyone who is a parent or who has a child in their life has experienced this. I'm a parent. I have two adult children. But throughout their entire lives, and even to this day, I write their future stories in my mind. Who do I want them to be? Who will they become? What amazing things will they accomplish, and what will my existence mean to them?

There comes a time in life when people want to write their own stories. At the end of life, I meet many people who want more time to write, who aren't ready to put the pen down, who feel that they have more to accomplish. I also meet people who are prepared and ready for the end; they are resigned to the finality of life and accept this natural course.

Spiritual Connection

My perspective on spirit involves distillation. The way I distill the concept of life is through the spirit. That nonphysical part of us, that essence of being. The spirit is our animation, and in some cultures, it is our breath.

There's an ancient Hebrew word called *ruha*, meaning breath.[11] A newborn breathes in for the first time upon being born; and upon the end of life, that last breath will be taken. The breath bookends life.

We have this spirit that isn't visible, but we know that it is there. It is like wind. We feel a breeze, we see the effects of it, but we don't see the wind itself. It is my belief that the spirit is this way. I often see the spirit manifesting itself through the energy of emotions and personalities. I am the keeper of this spirit, of the fear, anxiety, hope, anger, or joy that a person may have during their hospitalization.

I can empathize and reflect on the emotions, helping people to find their resiliency even with illness or injury. I listen to their thoughts of how they perceive illness or how they envision recovery. I can see how the spirit, that essence of being, manifests energy, emotions, inner thoughts, or outward personality. I can also see the essence of the spirit through character, ethics, morals, the things that matter most; through culture or religion; or through the things that make that person unique. That's my connection as chaplain.

That concept of human connection cannot be minimized. We thrive with human connection. We need a friend who lights up our energy and incites a hug, feeding that energy between us. We seek that spiritual energy of love, of affection, of connection, of thought whether we are sick or well.

Spirit connects us to something greater than ourselves, something transcendent, which could be religion, tradition, or spirituality. It could be God. It could be anything greater than the issue at that moment. Illness and injury are big. Many people who are sick or in a hospital are looking for something bigger than themselves, bigger than their illnesses, to hold on to, to put their faith into, and to support them while they go through this thing. They go to something that is transcendent.

I also pray with people. I do this to connect them with something that is greater than them. I may do rituals with them to bring them into that sense of transcendence. The spirit has a lot of different manifestations.

Take, for example, Agnes. I asked her about her family and what it was like when she was growing up. I wanted to learn about her. She was messing with me and teasing me. She was busting my chops. She said, "I was my mom's favorite." I got her sense of humor right away. I got the essence of her spirit through her humor. And I chuckled, and I thought it was wonderful. But it was just that moment when I got a sense of who she was.

And it wasn't just that. It wasn't just in her humor. It was how she cared for people, how she used her intelligence, how she connected with people, and how she remembered the names and stories of everyone who cared for her. Her tribe was very important. She was a respected elder in her tribe. She was a veteran in the locker room. And she was the one who had accumulated wisdom to give to others. She still had chapters to live out, but she wanted to bust my chops, and I got a sense of her spirit through that. I also got to pray with her.

In prayer, I want to connect with people. I want to know who they are. I seek to understand the essence of the individual, whether it's their sense of humor, their personality, what they want for themselves, how they handle rough and tough situations, or how I can support them during their recovery. I am not just looking at quantitative outcomes. I am not just looking to help them add to their years. I am looking for qualitative outcomes. I want their years to be good years.

I want to hear who they are in their own story. Are they a hero in their story? A villain? Are they a person who runs and hides, or are they the one who goes to the front of battle when the battle is getting hot? I want to know their identity, their role in life. Who are they as a spouse, a brother, a sister, a grandparent? What lights them up? What is the life-giving force that they have? I want to know what their identities are, and then I want to hear the stories because that's where the good stuff is—that's the connection and the meaning of their life.

I went into this room. The patient was an eighty-year-old gentleman named Max, and he needed surgery. He was laying in his bed and had a serene look on his face, and his granddaughter was at the bedside holding his hand, doing kangaroo care and stroking his head. His daughter and his son were seated on the back couch, all of them together as several generations of family who loved and supported each other.

His granddaughter started telling me who he was. He had to get some things taken care of health-wise, and I listened to him and his family tell the stories. He was a woodworker his whole life, and now that he was in his later years, he made objects for his family and friends. That was his love language. So, just like Agnes's love language was the way she manifested her spirit through knowing people's names and knowing what they were doing to help care for her, Max's was a spirit of creativity where he whittled things for people. He gave people things. He had a spirit of generosity and creativity. I was fascinated by the stories that his family told me about what he did and who he was.

Like Agnes, he had a sense of humor, and his manifested as dad jokes. I know those too well, according to my children. But he would tell these little dad jokes, and his grandchildren were like, "Oh, he's going to teach us how to do handstands." They each showed me pictures of how he had helped them to do handstands when they were kids; it was his way of "turning their world upside down" or "showing them a new perspective." They described him as having an encouraging spirit. Each one of them told me stories about when life hadn't gone right, and they'd needed someone to encourage them. Max had been that encourager.

And I was suddenly getting the essence of Max's story. By listening to his identity, and by listening to the stories, I was getting a sense of what the meaning and purpose of his life was and what this meant for him. I understood what this health situation meant for him and in terms of our mission as a team at Generational Health. He wanted to recover to continue his part of the story with his family, and he wanted more memories. He had more chapters to write.

Loving Life

I like to sail. My wife and I have been sailors for years, and we have friends who sail. We went to the British Virgin Islands in the Caribbean Sea in January of 2024. I had sailed on lakes and in San Diego Bay, but getting into the ocean was a different situation. There were different currents, different obstacles, and different wind. The wind shifted in different ways on the ocean, creating new challenges.

It was similar to what happens when someone gets into the later years of their life. They had been a seasoned captain of their own life. They may have sailed many seas or written many chapters. But now the current is different. The winds are changing, and the obstacles are new. In sailing, it is not about how you get into a situation. It is about how you get through it. It is about resiliency. Being in new seas—with changing winds, currents pulling in new directions, unanticipated obstacles, or a need for navigation—is what our patients face. Hopefully, through our work, we reflect the good parts, the memories, and the positive emotions, and they can better navigate with us behind them, lifting them up and supporting them until they find their own way.

—John, chaplain (San Diego, California)

A cancer diagnosis becomes the central focus of a person's life, often for months or even years during treatment. It's impossible to receive that diagnosis and then simply return to life as it was—the diagnosis is a pivotal event that changes everything. That moment will be forever etched in the patient's memory, and it carries a tremendous responsibility for our team. We value our ability to be compassionate during that time, and we recognize that our role is crucial in shaping the patient's experience with this life-changing information.

In oncology, we often see patients accompanied by multiple generations. Many are caring for young children or aging parents while dealing with their own illnesses. I think about that often—how spent I felt while embedded in the sandwich generation for my family, and how I didn't have the burden of critical or terminal illness. I want to find ways to alleviate that pressure from my patients.

—Gina, oncology director (San Diego, California)

Grace was seventy-two and had undergone an elective operation. She and her husband had thought that the procedure would be straightforward, so they'd sought out a surgeon in their favorite vacation spot, thinking to hit two birds with one stone. There was a surgical complication that took months to heal and required another operation. The second surgery was difficult, but it was able to be successfully completed, and the team was hopeful that she would start to recover. About three weeks into that recovery, though, she started vomiting and she couldn't stop. CT scan imaging showed a large mass in her pelvis, something that had not been seen six weeks prior when she had undergone a work-up and preparation for the second operation. The mass was a large, aggressive, rapidly growing cancer—and her life expectancy was on the order of a few weeks.

All she wanted to do was go home, back to a different state, where her family and friends were. Her husband wanted to support her in this, but he also wanted to be safe. He wanted to be able to provide the necessary care, and that meant getting her onto a plane and completing the trip. But he wasn't in perfect shape, either.

She required full nursing support for everything. She was too weak to walk, too weak to bathe, and too fatigued to do anything. She was dying. He carried the burden of telling her that she was never going to go home again. It may have broken both of them—being in a place that wasn't home, going through the end of her life together, and him ultimately making that return trip without her and walking into their home without her.

The more I thought about it and the more I heard from nurses, the less I could be present for them. I found that I couldn't walk into her hospital room. I couldn't face her, him, or what I knew was happening. I couldn't face the reality of her situation and what she wanted most, how I knew that level of yearning to be home, or how sick she was and how quickly she was declining. I couldn't be there. And I felt incredibly guilty about feeling this way. To this day, I wonder if that was how they remembered me.

People at the hospital who knew me and knew the situation understood how stressful it was to watch someone deteriorate so quickly and how hard that was as a physician who was there for healing. I didn't quit, and I had to remind myself of that. I recognized where the stress of caring for someone was overwhelming, and I took a step back. It was acceptable to admit this. There were plenty of other people who could take on the emotional burden and provide respite for me. It was similar to how caregivers felt at times—they loved the person, but it was normal to experience fatigue from the care. It was OK to need a break. It was healthy to care for myself and to allow others to pick up where I could not.

—Anonymous, primary care physician (Houston, Texas)

Before I was in Generational Health and Advanced Illness Management, I was a trauma nurse. I also worked in hospice, and before that, I studied religion and psychology. All of the elements that I've encountered in people have shaped my thinking and reinforced that every moment makes a difference in some spiritual way.

I joke that my soul age is ninety-five, so that's where my brain tends to go. I am an old soul in how I view connection and its imprint on the path of life, shaping the future trajectory, whether positively or negatively. Every person has a story, and every story comes from the journey, challenges, or miracles of life that have made some emotional impact. The stories about the journey of life are the most interesting and fascinating.

My grandmother lived her whole life in Central Park South in New York City. She was a diehard Yankees fan, which is why I am now rooting for the Yankees even though I'm not a baseball enthusiast. She had a heart-shaped framed picture of Derek Jeter in her apartment. I grew up staring at him and understanding the importance of baseball in her life.

She was a volunteer at Lenox Hill Hospital for thirty-five years, and they all knew her. When I started nursing school, and later on this path, I thought of her volunteering and what it meant to her. Her time was a gift she gave to the sick and injured. I love older adults and the aging population, which makes me think of her. Her legacy was in shaping the lives of people who weren't feeling well. She would visit them and talk about baseball. The magic was deception. She would steer clear of the obvious topics of disease and hospitalization, and would instead focus on baseball, a level playing field where people could forget about being sick. She was philanthropic with her time, highlighting how modern and interesting she was in doing things that were novel and completely selfless.

When I think about the power of human connection, it is passion and magnetism that create energy, momentum, and sustenance. It was my grandmother's strength and confidence that drove her to volunteer, to love strangers, and to give a piece of herself to people who were hurting. I constantly hone my memory of her strength. When I am trying to build my confidence, I say I am going to be like Nannie today.

I am an expert at end-of-life care, and I spend my work life with people who are facing end-of-life and their families. My interactions with patients are at times limited, a snapshot of whatever moment I am experiencing with them at the hospital. I think about our conversations, the snippets of their lives that they want to share with me at the end. I carry those pieces with me, and they impact my story. Telling the stories of loved ones is the epitome of their ethereal existence, a mechanism to keep the memories alive and to keep the energy relevant and active.

There was a Generational Health patient who was preparing for surgery, and she told me how she loved vacationing with her friends. Her biggest goal, and what mattered most to her, was going to New Orleans. I told her that I really would love to travel, but because I have a two-year-old, I have put traveling on hold for a bit. She kept telling me, "You got to go. You got to go." Because of something about her energy in that moment, I believed her. I was facing a once-in-a-lifetime opportunity to join a wellness retreat. It was out of town, and I had reliable care for my toddler. It was OK for me to travel, and I could leave him safely and still experience things. There was no reason for me to wait on him to grow up before allowing myself to have experiences of my own. Her influence was her legacy to me.

Another thing I know from my end-of-life care is that a single moment of time is enough to make an impact. I feel privileged to get that glimpse into someone else's life. Every so often in taking care of someone, I get to be a part of a time that matters, and I get to hear about a cherished moment from someone's childhood or a significant memory. Especially in my role in Advanced Illness Management, when we are discussing end-of-life decisions or really challenging decisions, I get to understand people. I get to understand their beliefs, their cultures, and their values. I am invited to understand their limitations, their humanity, and how it looks to consider all options. Some people have a strong character or an inner strength that absorbs pain or suffering. They wear it on the inside to not burden their loved ones, but those are the people who speak to my soul, my inner Nannie. She prepared me to recognize those who value strength and to support them with my whole heart in times of adversity.

An ideal experience for a patient considers all of these things and puts the patient at the center. It includes them in the conversation and ensures understanding. It is also a feeling. An attitude. A culture. I have seen other professionals empower patients, and in a moment of medical importance, make them feel like they are the only person in the room. I try to emulate that, as I think that is one of the greatest qualities a provider can have.

Patience in health care is also a tremendous gift. When you are in a rush, patients can feel that—and if you are in a rush to get to the next task, then you will miss the story. You will miss the legacy, the good stuff. While you may get the gist of the medical issue, you will miss everything else that makes that person special and gives them value.

—Jill, advanced illness nurse (San Diego, California)

Advocacy

Health-care providers are expected to be extraordinary, recognizing vulnerability and providing intentional expertise to push for the betterment of those they serve with directed purpose, consideration, and attention to detail and delicacy. To do this in the interest of a stranger, to invest heart and mind into another person who needs help, this is to have advocated for someone who may not have been able to do it alone.

MANY YEARS AGO, I completed the Camino de Santiago[12] in Spain. It was a journey of over 150 miles that culminated in me learning quite a bit about myself. The main lesson was the power of community. Throughout the entire hike I encountered villagers who fed me, other journeymen who needed camaraderie to continue forward, and all of my loved ones back home upon whom I relied to root me on and encourage me when I didn't think I could continue. On the very last day of the hike, when I knew I would reach the church, one of the friends I'd made along the way twisted her ankle. I wanted her to be a part of the end goal and get to the finish line. It was important to support her in getting to the church so that we could all complete the Camino together. That we could all share the energy and pride at the end of our journey together mattered to me. Finishing alone would have met the goal, but finishing with friends held an intangible value. I realized in that moment my ability to be present for others and my investment in other people's wins.

My dad had a chronic illness that he didn't understand, and because he didn't understand it, he couldn't speak for himself or ask important questions. He wasn't able to prepare. There was no plan B because there wasn't even a plan A. He needed an expert team that was invested in his well-being to guide him through the decision-making process. I also needed that; I needed to not be alone while dealing with my dad's care. I needed to be able to concentrate on supporting my dad instead of trying to figure out how to navigate the system. I was looking for a concept in medicine that was similar to my own journey on the Camino: people supporting people and caring about them getting to the finish line.

My dad had been living out of town when he was first diagnosed. I asked him to come to San Diego where I was living. He was my favorite person, and I wanted him to have the experience of community. I wanted him to feel supported.

There was a program called Generational Health that was dedicated to older adults and touted a "spectrum of care" for aging loved ones. I found the level of support that he needed with Generational Health. They helped coordinate the care. Behind the scenes, nurses, doctors, and skilled therapists were communicating about my dad. They were organizing the care and focusing on him and the things that were important to him. Within a week, he was started on a full-body program, chemotherapy, rehabilitation treatments, and overall lifestyle changes. He had a ready-made support system that was critical with a new, complicated, all-encompassing illness.

He never would have been able to navigate that alone. I also couldn't do it for him. This was new for both of us, and we didn't know what pathway to take. Generational Health provided what was needed, and we weren't encumbered with figuring it out on our own. We weren't alone in this fight anymore. We had a team, and that was the greatest part of the journey.

—David, dedicated family member (San Diego, California)

I finished four years in the marine corps with a slight sense of guilt at having spent a good amount of time away from my parents and grandparents. We were a close-knit family.

When my grandfather passed away from Parkinson's disease in 2022, I took a pause with my trajectory. I didn't have a clear next step, and my grandmother needed support. My grandma was going to adjust to a new life without my grandfather, and I didn't want her to feel alone. My grandfather ran the household business; the finances, the paperwork, and anything that needed annual renewal was his responsibility. Watching my grandmother try to navigate these things, I realized immediately that she couldn't do it without help.

Technology was moving at a pace where she couldn't keep up with it all. There were QR codes, websites, emails, clickbait, and bots, and it was so difficult to just get to a person and ask a question. She was lacking peer support and wanted to be online to make friends or catch up with long-lost ones. She hadn't grown up in a world with technology, and she hadn't had a regular need for the internet while my grandfather had been alive. He had navigated the world for her. She was vulnerable, and that vulnerability was attractive to strangers to take advantage of her. It angered me thinking of someone in the world trying to take advantage of my grandma and trying to rob her after she and my grandfather had lived their life together protecting their nest egg. This was a real motivator for me to stay on top of her online activity and to be involved in her business. She needed me, someone she trusted, to embark on that world for her and ensure her safety through basic daily internet interactions. She also needed teaching. She was cognitively intact and could learn to empower herself.

And then, one day, it hit me like a ton of bricks. She was one of millions of older adults who were probably facing the same challenge. I vividly remember her saying that despite all the new safety features programmed into cars these days, she felt less safe driving because she didn't know how to use them. This inspired me to make a difference in how seniors interact with technology.

—Cole, Senior Tech Connect,[13] (Oceanside, California)

I am a "born and raised" ED nurse. I started out as a technician in our ED in 2012, then went to nursing school and was hired as a new-grad registered nurse in our ED. Fast-forward ten years, and I am now an experienced ED nurse. In these last twelve years, I have participated in the care of thousands of patients from all walks of life, young and old, ranging from cardiac arrest and stroke patients to gunshot victims, to couples going through a miscarriage, to patients who have had toe pain for a few years and want to have it evaluated at three in the morning.

I have bonded with many amazing colleagues within my department who have become like family. I have had the time to educate myself about the many resources the hospital has to offer our patients and employees. I have also had the "privilege" of working on the front lines of a worldwide pandemic. So, with this work background of mine and knowing the stress the ED staff endure, I know how to laugh. I had a great sense of humor and a quick wit long before I honed them as my coping mechanisms. And that was because I inherited them from the even funnier person I was raised by: my father.

I am honored to share a bit about him. My dad, Bob (or, as he would introduce himself to my friends, "Bob with One 'o'"), was born in 1949 in Oak Ridge, Tennessee. You may recognize the name of that town from the recent movie, *Oppenheimer*[14] as it is the home of the Oak Ridge National Laboratory of the Manhattan Project.[15] The city was built basically from scratch in 1942, and my father's father (my grandfather) was recruited by the Manhattan Project to work at one of the plants in Oak Ridge to extract uranium for the atomic bomb. Granted, we later learned that neither he nor his coworkers knew what they were working to make. He met my grandmother around the same time, and she also worked at one of the plants. She was one of the "girls of Atomic City".[16] They started their family together, and this was where my aunt was born, followed by my father.

My grandfather died in 1961 at the age of thirty-nine of small bowel cancer when my dad was just eleven years old. My dad told me that he always wondered if his dad was proud of him, and he was worried—as an innocent eleven-year-old boy—that he never got to tell his dad how much he really loved him. He vowed at that point in his life to not let others—especially his future children—wonder the same. Years passed by, and my grandmother remarried a wonderful man when my dad was in high school, and my dad soon became incredibly close to his stepfather. My grampy—as I knew him—was diagnosed with pancreatic cancer in the late eighties, and his health declined rapidly. My dad saw the writing on the wall as his health worsened, that the end of his life was obviously nearing.

My dad, now an adult, remembering the feeling he had when he'd lost his father as a young boy, tried many times to talk to his stepfather about his treatment goals and his end-of-life wishes, while also trying to, most of all, make sure his stepfather knew how much he loved him. But Grampy was the ultimate optimist, never wanting to acknowledge how sick he was and never willing to talk about his wishes or say goodbyes. After Grampy died in 1991, my dad, yet again grieving a father, vowed a second time to not let others in his life wonder what his wishes were or wonder how he felt about them. He also never had the experience of helping his aging parents navigate plans for their last years of life as they faced terminal illnesses, and he didn't know what resources were available to help.

Now here are a few of the important CliffsNotes from the many years from then to now.

As a toddler, I lived full time with my dad. He was a doting thirty-five-year-old single dad trying to figure out how to raise an adorable three-year-old daughter. He soon married my beloved stepmom, and we all picked up and moved from Monterey, California, to a small town outside of San Luis

Obispo (SLO), California. I started kindergarten, and he started his financial planning business as a one-man shop. My brother arrived a couple years later, and he and I were raised by the most selfless, generous, hardworking parents in our tiny town outside of SLO.

My dad soon became a pillar in the community. He served on the board of Cuesta College[17] and Cal Poly,[18] was Rotary club[19] president, and was asked to speak and emcee at literally hundreds of community events as he had a knack for public speaking. He was a longtime member of the foundation for the local hospital, where my stepmom is still currently a thirty-plus-year active volunteer. And he was also on the board of SLO Hospice. His business flourished and became one of the biggest financial planning firms in the Central Coast. And throughout all this, he was the ultimate dad. He had no shame in crying in front of us, and he told us he loved us every day.

In the mid 2000s, my dad and my aunt were diagnosed with pulmonary fibrosis a few months apart. I cannot say for sure, of course, but the fact that they were both conceived, born, and raised in a city full of radioactive uranium may have had something to do with it. My aunt's disease progressed very quickly, and she received a double lung transplant, which gave her an extra ten years of life with her grandchildren before she died of unrelated causes in 2016. My dad's disease followed the status quo for about fifteen years, which baffled the experts, but we weren't complaining. He golfed four times a week, traveled the world, and lived his life to the fullest.

In 2020, I had my first real big brush with his mortality and the beginning of what would morph into the hard, bittersweet battle between being a knowledgeable, experienced nurse and a loving, scared daughter.

My dad was diagnosed with small bowel cancer in the summer of 2020 and needed to undergo surgery. In the weeks of planning before the surgery, which was happening during the early stages of a worldwide shutdown, I urged him to have it done at a bigger hospital in San Francisco, Los Angeles, or San Diego. I wanted him to be in a place with more resources for his lungs, in case they proved problematic during the operation. He was adamant about being close to home and wanting his surgeons, who were also his friends and fellow board members, as his teammates for this. There was a sense of pride in that—the hospital where he had been influential would now be caring for him. I found myself emotionally struggling because I knew how risky and complicated this surgery would be; and this was mixed with the fear of potentially losing my father (which was something none of us wanted).

My nurse brain and my daughter heart wanted to give him the best possible chance for survival and recovery. So, as he underwent his surgery there, I stayed in nurse mode; as one of the only medical experts in the family, I felt like I had to be. Someone had to be the medical advocate, the person to translate the medical jargon, the person to know the signs of deterioration, the person to ask the right questions, the person to keep him safe and healthy. This prevented me from being mentally present with my dad on the morning of his surgery. He sat next to me on the couch and told me how much he loved me, and that if something happened to him in the OR, that he was so proud of me. I just smiled and nodded and then told him to go take his pre-op shower.

He survived the surgery. But what was supposed to be a four- to five-day hospital stay turned into fifty-two days. He had post-op complications that required him to have drains hooked up to suction. This also meant he could not eat or drink the entire time to allow the bowel to heal.

Pandemic

But here was the kicker.

It was the summer of 2020. The policy at the hospital at the time was that one visitor was allowed at the bedside, but it had to be the same visitor for the entire admission. We obviously picked my stepmom to be that person because we thought he would be home in a couple days.

I know I was not the only one to miss being bedside with a loved one during the pandemic, and I have deep empathy for all who experienced that. It was quite the mind game to be the nurse screener standing in front of our ED turning visitors away all day long while seeing the anguish on their faces, and trying to console them. All the while I had also been turned away from seeing my dad.

When I would go up to visit, I would climb through the bushes on the side of the one-story hospital to his window and wave and do silly dances for him. I would wait at our house for my stepmom to come home with any pictures on her phone of the IV bags hanging, or of the plan on the whiteboard. Sometimes, a nurse would let her take a picture of the order screen on their computer. Because Lord knows, when I called my parents to ask for updates, I would get, "The surgeon came by and said things are going as planned. Oh, and the nurse just hung the bag of those fluids and gave him some medicine."

Cool. Helpful. Thanks.

I would troll his health app and read any progress notes I could. And when I had updates, I found myself quickly consulting with my colleagues to help me understand the results or vent about my frustration with his complications. They would hold space for me to freak out a little bit. The people I found myself talking to were the surgeons I worked alongside and my colleagues on our Generational Health team. And, in fact, it was one of those people, Kelly, who literally said, "Follow me," and brought me over to one of our surgical oncologists whom I had never met before. She said, "Tell him your story." He listened to me and kindly gave me some recommendations to suggest to my dad's medical team four hundred miles away. I did just that. And they listened and tried it. And it worked. My dad came home five days later.

Some may say this was just lucky because I worked in a hospital and had lots of medical friends and connections. That could be a little bit true. But I think it just comes down to knowing what resources you have available to you—as an employee at a hospital or as a nonmedical community member—and utilizing them. What I needed was someone objective, not someone who was emotionally connected to my father, to look at the situation and treat me like a family member and not like his nurse. Someone who could take that burden off of me.

When my dad came home, he still wasn't allowed to eat and had a PICC line[20] with daily infusions to manage for a couple more weeks. We knew home health was coming to visit, but I still took time off to go home and help out, mostly to give my stepmom a break. The home health nurse came the first day and showed us how to mix the IV bags and prime the lines.

I said, "Great. Thank you. See you tomorrow."

And she said, "Tomorrow? No, I just come once a week and bring you the week's supply."

"Um, what?"

It was at that moment that I quickly had to jump back into nurse mode and become Nurse Ratched[21] (as my dad started to call me then, and kept calling me for the rest of his life).

I managed his drips and his supplies, checked his vitals, etc. While my very sharp, educated stepmom would have figured it all out, she was beyond mentally and emotionally exhausted at that point. It was simply too much for her to continue to give care after a long, stressful hospital stay.

They needed help, and the only quick resource we had set up at that point in our small town was me. But I was more than happy to help. This was my specialty, and it was at times a fun way to show my parents what I actually did for a living. I saw them respect my medical knowledge more, and they may have realized that I knew what I was talking about. The flip side was that I didn't get to relax much and just be with my dad. I couldn't turn my nurse brain off.

I was Nurse Ratched, not daughter Stef.

No matter how much I tried to mentally hand off the nursing burden I felt, it stayed (or maybe it was scarier to just let it go).

He fully recovered from that a couple months later, and life got back to normal. Golf, travel, work, and grandkids. Life was good.

In the fall of 2022, my dad came down to San Diego with a few of his buddies for a Padres game. I met up with them for dinner and noted that my dad had labored breathing and was lethargic.

Nurse Ratched activated.

I told him I was taking him to *my* ED, and I wasn't giving him a choice. I said, "Get in the car. You're in *my* house now."

Being in Control

He was admitted for his upper respiratory infection for a couple days, and while things forever changed for him after that episode, I am so glad it happened while he was here in San Diego. In those couple days, I was able to just be at his bedside and be his daughter. I knew his medical team was top-notch because I had an established relationship with them, and I was able to tap into the resources to get him set up to get back home. We all felt more relaxed and supported. He went home on oxygen from that admission and never got off of it again.

Through the rest of 2022 and then into 2023, his pulmonary fibrosis progressed rapidly. Now that he was sick enough to qualify for a transplant, he was too old at seventy-three. He quickly went from walking around on a small amount of portable oxygen, still golfing and working, to not being able to walk from the house to the garage without resting. He was unable to emcee events because he couldn't catch his breath.

By the late part of 2023, he had to use a wheelchair to get anywhere and had maxed out on the amount of oxygen any home device service could deliver. His local medical team consisted of his concierge doctor, and that was about it. His local pulmonologist had retired. He relied upon one internal medicine doctor to manage all of this, and while she was great, it wasn't working for his needs. Nobody was educating him on titrating his oxygen usage or supplies or things to look out for.

So here came Nurse Ratched again, being the oxygenation educator and supply purchaser, the lab work interpreter, the "what dose of pain meds should I take today" teller, etc. He didn't want to tap into any other local resources because, honestly, he didn't know what he didn't know.

Thankfully, he had been seen at UCSF Lung Clinic[22] many years prior, so we reached out to them for him to be seen again. We all went to his appointment where, by no mistake, he was "randomly" assigned to a pulmonologist who specialized in end-stage disease. She spent an hour with us, explaining the disease process and his poor prognosis. She referred him to palliative care, which my parents had never heard of.

Palliative care was something I had known about from my work with Generational Health, but it was not mainstream in my dad's small town.

Palliative care allows you to continue to seek curative treatment but aims to sustain your comfort and quality of life.

The palliative care referral was not only the best thing for my dad at that point, but it was a great relief to me. In fact, the pulmonologist called me out of the blue the next day after that first appointment just to check on me and to promise me that I would not have to be the one to have the hard discussions about end-of-life with my dad. She said she could tell my parents were not quite ready to hear all of the options just yet, and that was OK. She knew from the look on my face that I knew where this was all headed. That it would keep progressing fast, and that he most likely would not make it to my brother's wedding in May. She told me that she saw the nurse in me and the daughter in me, and she wanted to lift that burden. It was her job, and she promised to take some of that off my shoulders so I could grieve and be with my dad during these last months of his life.

That was the first time I cried.

On the phone to a random pulmonologist I'd just met the day before.

I finally had help. I finally had a plan. I didn't have to hold all the weight.

Our appointments with palliative care were helpful, and my parents even began to talk in lighter tones of voice because they finally felt supported and seen. They had help. My dad was asked what parts of his life were most important, and he said he wanted to be with his family and friends as much as possible, and not undergo tons of doctors' appointments. He wasn't ready to stop any treatments. We focused on that. Not only did the palliative care doctor hear those answers, but we all heard them, so we knew what was important to him. We even figured out how to get a couple of small tanks and thirty feet of tubing on his golf cart so he could cart around with his friends and hit a few balls.

For me, there was an initial sense of relief from having palliative care involved.

But then things got worse.

My nurse anxiety began to grow as his health progressed. He had said many times that he wanted to die at home. He did not want to be poked and prodded in a hospital.

In my time as an ED nurse, I have seen more than my fair share of chronically ill, end-of-life patients come in receiving CPR, with us pounding on their chest, having breathing tubes put down their throat, putting them on ventilators, and poking them with needles as their family waited in agony because they'd never discussed end-of-life wishes with their loved one and now, at the hardest moment, they didn't know what to do.

I have also seen families bring in actively dying loved ones who have had those discussions about not resuscitating them, and I have been able to provide comfort and peace and hold space for those people as they passed the way they wanted to.

I wanted my dad to start hospice so that logistics and do not resuscitate (DNR) orders would be in place. I wanted to make sure that medications would be at the house, a nurse would be on call if something happened, and there would be a plan that honored my dad's wishes to die at home. And when he lost his decision-making abilities and mental faculties, my stepmom would be empowered to follow those plans.

I was terrified that he would fall or get a fever or go into respiratory distress, and that my stepmom would have to call 911, and he would end up at the hospital being poked and prodded and would never come home. I knew all the medical things that could happen; and without hospice set up, the likelihood of those things happening was much greater than his wishes of dying peacefully at home. I tried to explain my reasoning to convince my parents to enroll. But the decision wasn't up to me.

In January, we went to another appointment at UCSF, and that pulmonologist told him that it was time to start hospice. My dad said that while a part of him knew it was time, he didn't want to "give up."

This is a common misconception, and there is a stigma about hospice—especially in the older generations. To many, hospice is synonymous with death. It is thought to mean you've given up and gone home to die. It is seen as someone lying unconscious in a bed, with no quality of life; when, in reality, it is care for all different stages of the end of life. It is comfort care to go about doing activities that give you meaning and dignity. It is caregiver respite. It is a support group. It is social work. It is knowledgeable providers who care for patients at the end of life.

It is *not* giving up.

It is taking control of how you want to live out the last months of your life. But, at the same time, it is the hardest pill for patients and families to swallow, to accept that death is coming. I get that. And with my dad, as I sat in that appointment with the blank POLST[23] DNR forms, he was trying to simply accept that it was his time.

As he put it, "I'm not scared of dying. I'm just not anxious to."

We left that appointment *not* enrolled in hospice. My nurse brain was so scared for him while my daughter heart was so scared for *me*.

As we got in the car, my parents asked my brother how he was feeling, and they asked each other what they felt. But nobody asked me what I felt because, as my brother said, "We know you're fine; you deal with this every day." It was like I had been in Nurse Ratched mode for so long that my parents had forgotten I was a daughter with feelings about my dad dying.

There I was, trying to convince my dad to enroll in hospice so he could die the way he wanted to, but also trying to accept the mere fact that my dad was dying.

It was at this point when I reached out to Generational Health to ask for help. I asked for help for what to say to my parents to help guide them in their decision. To my surprise, the nurses and doctors on the team kindly offered to sit in on meetings with my dad as a third party so that I, his daughter, wasn't the one explaining it to him again. I think everyone could see the turmoil I was experiencing as a nurse-daughter. In hindsight, I wish I would have reached out to them earlier in the process to lighten the load on me, a heavy load I didn't even fully realize I had been carrying.

A couple weeks later, in early February, my brother and his fiancée threw a last-minute wedding in the backyard of my parents' house. It was just their immediate families, so my dad could see his baby boy get married. My dad was beaming in his favorite suit that was now way too big for him on his frail body. He gave his planned champagne toast in our living room. He truly never stopped smiling the whole day. It was a stark reminder to me to slow down and be present. To stop. To let Nurse Ratched go for the short time I had left with him and just be *with* him.

He enrolled in hospice on Tuesday. The nurse met him on Wednesday, and all the logistics were set, with medications in the house and phone numbers to call on the fridge by Thursday. My parents had a good, long cry but felt good with the plan that was now in place. In fact, my dad didn't even text me until Friday night to say, "Oh, by the way, hospice is all set up and good to go. Love ya!"

After all that … by the way!

Peace

On Sunday, he had his best friend over to the house, had a barbecue, and watched his beloved 49ers lose the Super Bowl. On Monday, he was sitting at his desk working on some spreadsheets when he suddenly felt tired and laid down on his favorite couch that overlooked the bay. He became confused, and his oxygen saturation plummeted. A week earlier, my stepmom would have had to call 911. But this time, she knew, even in her fear, to call his personal doctor and the hospice nurse. The doctor came over and helped her administer some of those new hospice meds to make him comfortable and breathe more easily. The doctor then told her to call me and my brother.

As I stood in the trauma room at work answering that call, I simply asked, "Do I need to come home?"

The doctor said, "Yes, you do," in the way that only fellow nurses and doctors understand the true meaning.

I knew I had to get the four hundred miles home as quickly as I could. I knew he was dying, but I wanted to make sure he really was comfortable, get him more meds, and take care of him one last time.

He died an hour before I got home and fifteen minutes before my brother got there. He peacefully passed away with my stepmom by his side, in the still of the night, on his favorite couch overlooking his favorite view.

Just the way he'd wanted.

When I walked in and saw him so peaceful, I felt the weight of the world lift off my shoulders. I was almost happy even, as weird as that sounds.

I also realized that, in the end, my dad had protected me. He'd known that I would have come in hot, asking what meds had been given and being the ultimate nurse at his deathbed. He'd died before I got there so that I could come in and be daughter. So I could hold my dad's hand and kiss him goodbye. It was his last way of thanking me and protecting me.

These last nine months without my dad still don't feel real. I realized what amazing gifts he'd given me and what I hoped to teach others from his story. Because of the losses he'd experienced early in life, he chose to talk about the hard things so they weren't hard to talk about. We talked a lot about death, what he hoped that would look like for him, what was important to him, and what he wanted for us. He set an example to hold space for the hard days and the good days, and to not lose sight of what filled my heart. I asked my stepmom recently if she had anything to add to this chapter, and she quickly said she wished they'd enrolled him earlier. She then told me how she was looking into hospice for my ninety-eight-year-old grandmother. Something she never would have considered before.

—Stef, emergency department nurse (San Diego, California)

Giving Back

To give of yourself, to share your experience or your expertise with others in a way that fosters learning or betterment of a situation, and to support growth through philanthropy of your time or your expertise is to have blessed those around you with a gift that wouldn't exist without you.

A GREAT HEALTH-CARE SYSTEM includes accountability, respect for each other, a shared mission, and a shared vision on how we improve our communities. It enables daily activities and tasks to be designed in such a way that the job part feels like it is supposed to; it feels like taking care of people, rather than feeling like work.

—Bijal, nephrologist (San Diego, California)

My career as a nurse officially started fifteen years ago; however, health care was on my horizon from the time I was a child. I played every sport vigorously, with my whole heart, passion, and persistence. I was dedicated to each team, where I learned to practice and improve skills, be kind to others, lend a hand when someone fell, and be competitive. I learned effort, hard work, teamwork, and compassion as a young athlete.

My mother had a chronic illness from the time I was four. I saw the despair in her eyes with every appointment. Every time a doctor failed to find an answer, she wanted nothing but to have a diagnosis, to feel normal again, and to not be a burden for her kids. I understood firsthand what it meant to not have an answer to symptoms. I wanted to be a nurse to support people like my mom who were going through the worst times of their lives. My mom wasn't defined by her disease; she was a strong woman who worked through chronic pain and a life-altering autoimmune disease that was trying but could not defeat her spirit or her function.

As the years went on, I committed to health care. I wanted to be a nurse. I started as a nursing student and matriculated over time to become a nursing assistant, new graduate, clinical nurse, advanced clinician, and now a nurse manager. The oncology unit where I initially trained also functioned as a palliative care unit focusing on alleviating symptoms while patients pursued either aggressive treatments or comfort care. Palliative care emphasized dignity and peace during the transition to a comfort-focused plan at the end of life. It was on this unit where I became invested in patients and the people they were in their real lives outside the hospital. I learned maturity, dignity, understanding differences, and humility.

I was a healthy adult caring for people and their loved ones at their most vulnerable—their most ill, scared, grieved, and grieving—and they entrusted me with this responsibility. Each of my patients left memories and impacted how I compassionately cared for people. I learned that our trajectory is limited. I saw that people facing mortality will fight until there is no fight left. That often the inner strength is relentless until the end.

I left oncology after seven years of bedside experience for an opportunity with Advanced Illness Management. I learned how to communicate with people about their wishes, educate them about their options, and be an expert in a field that people once thought was terrifying. This team and others who embraced palliative philosophy broke the stigma, tore down the walls, and opened the gates for people's voices to be heard. These treatment plans prioritized what was of the highest value to the person receiving the treatment or intervention. This team was pivotal to change in the nursing culture, leading the way to identify early goals of care and instill confidence in our expertise for the people receiving care.

Now, as a nurse, I welcome other people to lean on my strength when they can't find theirs. I hope I can rely on others in my time of need. Throughout my career, I have been grateful for the mentors and people who have been paired with me to teach, precept, and show me the ropes.

I am also fortunate to have a career rooted in caring for others at the hardest times of their lives while focusing on listening to them and collating what matters most to them into a functional and workable health-care plan. When I was a bedside nurse, I valued my time with patients who had been hospitalized for the fifth month in a row. I learned about their families and their lives outside the hospital. I was invested. I wanted to know who they were. While the phrase "what matters most" seemed obvious, it was often not considered in any nationally tracked health outcome. I felt responsible for ensuring that my philosophy and practice prioritized what mattered to my patients, but I also instilled that same attitude in my family and myself. I could only be my best for someone else if I treated myself with the same appreciation, gratitude, and grace I hoped my patients experienced in my care.

Going forward in this career, I want to innovate and find motivation in new knowledge and processes. Most importantly I want to be a mentor, an adviser, and a leader to others. I look forward to the future, knowing it could end at any moment—seconds, minutes, hours, or decades from now. I want to bring as much healing, health, and sustained happiness for however long my path will last.

—Kelly Wright (San Diego, California)

In 2013, I had a major fear of the unknown. I was working in my clinic when I started feeling flu-like symptoms that were persistent. The symptoms got worse. After several days in bed, my wife took me to the ED where I was found to have an illness that no one could figure out. No one could diagnose the cause.

In the next twenty-four hours, I did my best to try to die.

I had multi-organ failure. My heart was affected, and my kidneys were affected. I was confused, and I was at the hospital where I had been working as a physician leader for the previous six years.

There were upward of forty physicians, countless nurses, other specialists, and ancillary staff who supported me through that process of hospitalization. Their efforts for me, for my life, can only be described as the cutting edge of humanity.

I ended up in the ICU for about a week.

I was in the hospital for three weeks.

It took me about three months before I could walk. It took me a year to come back to work. It took me four years to fully recover.

I had something called streptococcal toxic shock syndrome with myositis and fasciitis, a severe, flesh-eating bacteria of my leg.[24] That was my fear of the unknown. I didn't completely understand what was happening to me, my life, my body, my future, and my family. And when you are sick, nothing else matters.

Confucius said (2,500 years ago, so it hasn't changed much): A healthy man wants a thousand things. A sick man only wants one.[25] That was how I felt. Suddenly, every previous magnanimous decision was fairly mundane, and the only thing that mattered to me was getting back to health. The team allowed me to take a shower about two and a half weeks after I'd first become ill. A real shower, not one in a bed. As the hot water hit me, I couldn't tell tears from the spray. Something I had taken for granted my entire life was my reality and became something overwhelmingly appreciated. That I could shower. That I could do it. And how much I needed that feeling of being clean. And how small of a need that was, but how real that feeling was in that moment. I only cared about getting better. I only cared about my family. I only wanted to survive.

I had that crash course at the young age of thirty-nine.

I'm fifty-one now, but that experience framed how I thought about life and how I thought about taking care of people. My own experience changed me. It changed me in the way I looked at physicians and nurses, and it helped me to focus on what was most important, which was relationships.

Connections and relationships saved my life. For the six years that I'd worked at the hospital and in the community,

I'd made connections and relationships with people, and I'd never realized or appreciated what that investment would ultimately bring. People made the difference of survival for me, but the investment on my end had been made before my illness. I was always polite and friendly with the entire team, the housekeeping staff, our volunteer services, other physicians, the concierge team, and others. When I was sick, these same people went above and beyond for me and continue today to check in with me and ask me how I am feeling.

And that came from me doing something as little as making a connection. All that self-talk was a reality for me through the dedication of others. That someone cared about me; that I was going to keep fighting.

Those moments were critical for me. Those moments pushed me forward.

I didn't need an endless network of strangers; I needed the people I regularly interacted with—my colleagues and peers. They were connected to me well enough to feel impacted by my story, to personalize my experience, and to root for me. I thought about this often in the context of personal space, and what was within and not within my control. In all the space where I was in control of my own decisions, I chose whether to be on display. I chose to prioritize how I looked to others or how I made other people feel.

Social media and technology have hugely impacted the world since the time of my illness more than ten years ago. I now realize that if I had been ill during the era of Facebook or Instagram, the messaging may have changed my experience, my recovery, and my impact on others. Although social media had its benefits, it also affected human connection, making it more impersonal for mass appeal. The way I connected with people, and the way I wanted them to connect with me, went beyond mere impressions or likes on a post. I experienced the true necessity of human connection, and it was the cutting edge of humanity.

Before my illness, I felt like, *Man, I am turning forty this year. It is terrible, I am getting old.* Eight months after my illness, I got to turn forty. And that was the thing: I got to turn forty. I was in bonus time. Every day that I lived after that illness was a chance to say to myself, *Gosh, this is pretty cool. I don't have to be here.*

After my illness, I asked myself, *What am I going to do with this knowledge, this experience of what I have gone through?* This question became my life's thesis. I was alive, and I was healthy. And what was I going to do with it? It was a gift, and I felt compelled to pay it forward.

I took inventory of my life: I was privileged, my parents loved me, I had a wonderful family, and I had supportive friends. Many of my patients never had a fraction of what I had, and I owed them the gifts that I had to give. I knew firsthand what it meant to have a support system while I was sick. I needed to give this back to others.

In my culture, age represented wisdom. An older relative was revered for their lifetime of achievement, rather than seen as a drain or a burden. Many families continued to dwell together, multiple generations, giving the children opportunities to bond with their grandparents and leverage those relationships to teach humility, respect, and appreciation. When I considered my own experience in the family unit in Pittsburgh, Pennsylvania, where I grew up and engaged in our health-care system, I saw the reemergence of elder appreciation through a health-care program that provided dignity in sickness or injury.

I related this bigger picture, this influence I was able to affect, and this concept of a timeline to the lessons I taught my children. I wanted them to follow my footsteps in one way: to use their privilege to better the world around them in a way that was meaningful to them, that carried purpose and respected the value of time. I told them that it was a gift to be privileged, and with that gift came responsibility. I showed them how to use their blessings to help underserved and underrepresented people. I also tried to provide them with a home that was seen as their refuge, the place where they could create freely and be themselves, and learn and grow without any negative influence. I wanted them to see the home as the place where they were valued and where they valued the older family unit.

My family wrote a mission statement, and we put it on a board in front of our house. It read: To gain knowledge and strength through study and experience while laughing along the journey, in an effort to support our friends and our family, to serve society. This mission was Polaris, our North Star. Something of value to hold when there was conflict or when life wasn't working out. My family provided this value. This was a life lesson that my family held dear, and it was an anchor for my children whenever they were unsure. That was the cutting edge of humanity. I wanted to be cutting-edge, and I wanted to show my children a way to use privilege to positively affect others. I wanted to give back.

In the context of power and long-term outlook, I thought about legacy for myself and for my family. In health care, short-term outcomes were appreciated and were the metrics used to justify success. A treatment led to an outcome, and that equaled merit. Weren't there long-term considerations that needed to be made to ensure sustainability?

I went back on to the lecture circuit sometime after my illness. I would talk about my journey, and people would come up to me afterward and say that I should go around the country sharing my story. And while I appreciated the compliment, I didn't imagine that would bring the type of fulfillment I was seeking. I would be connected to strangers for the moments of my talk, and then it would be over. I would be in a hotel, not knowing anyone, and then I would go home. And I would have missed that time with my wife and my children and my friends. And was that how I wanted to share this story of my experience of survival? Was that the meaning of my life that I wanted to share?

Especially when I was thriving on borrowed time, that concept didn't seem to jive with what I wanted.

I was left with the same questions: *What do I do now that I am recovered and have had this experience? How do I impact others in a way that is meaningful?*

I was still a nephrologist working with a large, multidisciplinary group practice. I became a partner in the organization, and I thought, *You know what? I want to build an economic engine or a business that is sustainable and lasting that can continue to provide for generations to come. If I just go and give talks and inspire a few people for a day, that won't do it. What if I build something with other people that continues to give so that there is sustainability and a legacy even after I die?*

I had something real to give.

I had been overseeing home dialysis in our group for nephrology patients since 2008, but I wanted to go farther and build more with them. I started doing things to help our patients and doctors.

In 2020, I decided that I was a little short on some of the education and the knowledge that I needed, so I pursued a master's degree in business.[26] I did this part time during COVID-19. The inflection point for me was a class called Power and Politics. Before taking this class, I had been of the mindset that people who craved power probably should not be in power. There seemed to be a disqualifier in having an intense need or want for power. Before this class, I'd felt like I would do good and powerful things, but only outside of the limelight. In this class, I learned that to be powerful you have to have power within; there had to be a need, a drive, a motivation. There was an opportunity to be chairman of the board in our nephrology group, and this was when I felt empowered to take on this responsibility on a greater scale. I was motivated for change, and I possessed the authority to institute positive change for our patients and their caregivers.

Caregiver support in nephrology was invaluable and could not be overlooked. In nearly all cases in our clinics, caregivers accompanied patients to their appointments. Often, these caregivers were family members or friends, not professionals or hired employees, providing compassionate support. What often went unnoticed was that caregivers may not have been working, as their time was devoted to providing care at home, potentially neglecting their own self-care.

It was easy to rush through appointments and forget that caregivers were integral to the patients' success, especially for nephrology patients who often progressed to end-stage disease and required substantial home support. Caregivers dedicated their lives to managing this medical condition and deserved to be included in the care plans they helped implement. They needed a voice, which was frequently overlooked in a system focused on task completion and quick appointments rather than person-centric care. In my role as chairman of the board, I was able to realign caregiver goals with our care model. I was able to bring the caregivers back to the center of the plan, making them just as critical as the patients we served.

My team was also able to pursue durable change by enabling free transportation for our renal patients who were often traveling to their appointments, to dialysis multiple times per week, and to the various specialists for routine follow-ups. It was eye-opening to find that there were patients who had appointments five miles from their homes, and they were reliant on a two-hour bus transportation to get them there. These determinants of health were critical to consider while trying to enact change.

About a year ago, it struck me that our greatest competition was not another hospital system; it was kidney failure. And if the competition was kidney failure, then the goals for how to combat it and how to make the care more efficient and patient-friendly were no longer elusive. It was easiest to fight an enemy when that enemy was identified and had a name. In my own journey of evaluating my values and taking inventory, I needed to know what I was fighting against. For my patients, it was the same. We fought together and we won together.

One of the biggest lessons I learned from my illness was the power of saying no. I had to learn to say no to things I had always said yes to. When caring for others, it was easy to forget to say no. Most health-care providers were accustomed to saying yes. When considering leadership, it was just as important to recognize when a situation was best left to others as it was to know when I could create lasting change. Saying no wasn't a sign of weakness or complacency; it was an acknowledgment that I was enough to make a crucial contribution or decision. I was enough, and I could ask for help. And if I asked for help, I was deserving of help. And with that validation, I was able to give more of myself to those around me. I was able to support my patients and their families best when I acknowledged my own limitations and gave myself space to be human.

I just hope everybody has a wonderful day, and I'm just going to tell you if you haven't heard it today: I love you.

—Bijal, nephrologist (San Diego, California)

I am primarily a volunteer. I've been volunteering with Sharp HealthCare for twelve years and am now with hospice services. Sharing my story about how I became a caregiver and then a volunteer feels so comfortable now, but when I started on this pathway, it was completely forced and unnerving.

As a teenager, I never wanted to be anywhere near a hospital. I didn't like going to the doctor. Everything about medicine was scary, painful, or confusing. To my dismay, I ended up having to become very involved in health care as a caregiver for my family, and then eventually for myself. What I found at the end of the road were all these wonderful people who spent their lives providing care, and many of them touched my life in some positive way.

My brother passed away from leukemia at the age of fifty-seven in 2012. He'd had a brain injury when he was eighteen months old. It was a very bad injury that caused him to have severe grand mal seizures for the rest of his life, and he was also developmentally delayed. He had to be cared for by my mother, who was a single mom. As a young teen, I helped her where I could, but then I was working, and then I was in the military for a while. When I came back, I began consistently helping her with his care. We did everything for him. He was completely dependent. We had to clean him and help him get up into a wheelchair from his bed. And as time went on, and my mother was getting older, I inherited more of these duties. This insidiously led to quite a bit of caregiving without me even realizing that was what I was doing. I was spending my time caring for my brother, providing around-the-clock homebound care. Then my mom got dementia, and she could no longer care for him at all, so I became his primary caregiver as well as hers.

To really understand the depths of caregiving, you have to understand the uncomfortable and difficult parts. If you know anything about dementia, you may know that sometimes the patient is incontinent. And that means that they'll just go whenever the urge comes. I was already helping my brother with his toileting, for which we had a pretty good routine. I would help him get in there with his wheelchair and transfer over. He would do his thing, then I would transfer him back. We had it down. Then my mom, with her dementia, needed that same level of care. And the thought of it … well, it was like a cartoon, really. I would be helping him, and then I'd hear her. "Wait, Mom!" I'd see her with her walker, and I'd have to chase her down the hall, hoping she wouldn't make any sudden moves, and then I'd run back to my brother. What a mess! Literally. I was like a ping-pong ball bouncing between them, and sometimes failing with both. I was drained.

We were in and out of the hospital for forty years as a family. As we did our back and forth, we became very close to many of the folks on the nursing units. They would see us time and time again because we were frequent fliers. I remembered the kindness and the calming effect of going into the hospital. I realized that many people who came into the hospital probably thought, *I'm going to be taken care of now*, or, *I am going to feel better now*. That stuck with me.

Then my mom passed away from dementia and complications from falling. And I asked myself, *What do I do now?* I had retired as a commercial industrial appraiser, and I had spent my available time in and out of the hospital caring for my family. I needed to do something with my life—and for the first time, I could do anything.

I was going to grief counseling because I was having a hard time dealing with my emotions. In one of the grief counseling sessions, there was a wonderful volunteer who talked about her marriage of sixty-two years to the love of her life. They'd both weathered the storm of losing their son when he was fifteen years old, and he had been their only child. She talked about being a caregiver over the last five years to her husband.

After he'd passed away, she'd asked herself, *What do I do now?*

I was immediately riveted by her story because I could completely relate. She went on to explain that her whole life had revolved around her husband—and before that, her child—and she didn't know what to do now that they were both gone. To manage her grief, she trained to be a hospice volunteer.

I listened to her speech, which was very inspirational. Afterward, I stopped her, and I said, "I would like to volunteer."

And she asked, "When did your family members pass?"

I replied, "It was about three weeks ago."

She said, "Well, you can't do that. You must wait a year. Deal with your own grief, and then come back to me."

I'd like to back up a bit about connection. Perhaps you have somebody in your life to inspire you, to move you, to cause you to want to live life. For the first part of my life, my brother and my mom filled these roles. But once they were gone, and I'd committed to volunteering, I was able to find that in the people I was helping.

I began my volunteer services as a community care partner, which is a person who dedicates a part of their day to supporting someone who is hospitalized. In the course of being a community care partner, I encountered many challenges with people. Some were very difficult. One of them, Ron, I remember vividly. He still visits the unit every year to thank the staff for their care.

Ron had stage four throat cancer when we first met. He was having a difficult time accepting what was going to happen to him. He was thinking there was not a whole lot of hope.

I introduced myself, and I said, "Well, would you like me to be your friend? I'm Gil." I then described how volunteers like me would visit daily.

He was confused, so I explained further. "Well, just because, you know, you look like you could use a friend."

He listlessly answered, "No, not today." He told me I could come back later if I wanted to.

And I kept going back. The next day, I went back in and visited with him.

"Oh, you're here again," he said. "No, I don't think I'm ready for it today."

Again, "No, I don't think I'm ready for it."

I skipped on with some other patients and then came back with another volunteer who was shadowing me. I said, "Hey, this is Rebecca. I want to introduce you. We are both here to help you."

And this time, he said, "OK."

"Persistent, at least," he said. "So what are you going to help me with?"

We were just going to talk and find out what his interests were. And while we did that, we were getting his confidence, and his understanding that we were there to listen. We were people who cared. He had been alone in fighting this alienating disease, spending considerable time in the hospital away from family or friends, and he was feeling irrelevant, as if the world had forgotten him. We were there to show him that he was important and that his life held meaning even while he was sick.

He liked art, so we engaged art therapy. Like magic, there was a change in the air, a lighter feel than what had been there before. The team was doing more than giving their time to a stranger; they were building a bond, they were building a network, and Ron didn't have to face the day-to-day in the hospital alone. I was also getting what I needed: that feeling of supporting someone else, that feeling of filling a void.

It turned out Ron was a pretty good artist. He started drawing various things that he would see every day at the hospital. He would sometimes draw pictures of the nurses and some of the adventures. These became gifts he could give away. He could leave a piece of himself with his care team. The days became shorter, more tolerable. We saw his visits as highlights in our schedule. He started talking to us about his cancer, about the things that mattered to him, and he asked us questions about life, death, and hope. His attitude became one of camaraderie rather than of defense. We felt we were making a difference for him. We were impacting his hospitalization in a positive way, but more importantly, he was teaching us about the power of community and the power of volunteerism and time. Time given to a stranger. It made a difference. It translated to caring. He wasn't alone. Ron continues to visit every year on the anniversary of his hospital discharge.

We moved on to patients in the trauma unit, and we were asked to help with a young lady who had told the nursing staff that she didn't think her life was worth living anymore. She didn't want to hurt herself, but she was severely depressed. She had been partying with friends, taken drugs, passed out, and woken up as a trauma patient. She told her nursing team that she felt like everyone in the world had dumped her. Her friends and her family had not visited, and no one was calling to check in. She felt alone and sad.

I came into her hospital room, and she said, "Why do you want to talk to me?"

"Well, I just think that you need a friend," I said.

"They won't let me have any of my old friends in here," she told me.

The medical team was trying to protect her.

My volunteer team talked to her, and there was a connection. Arts volunteers, musician volunteers, music therapists—we had a whole team of people coming in to see her, and we were her new friends. All of a sudden, she was telling us her story. It was difficult to hear. Her mother was a prostitute who had abandoned her. She started life out alone. She was put into foster care, which was dangerous for her, and she ran away. She was later taken in by people on the street. She had a hard time trusting that our team wanted to support her health journey. She rarely had a stable environment as a child, although there was one foster home where she'd learned art and music. This was a good memory that she shared with us.

The act of listening was powerful. Togetherness was power. She enjoyed music, so we wheeled her to the lobby where there was a pianist. She loved art, so we encouraged her to create. When people walked into her room, her paintings welcomed them. She had this bright light whenever any of us came into the room. Her whole attitude changed. She began to participate with her physical therapy. She was motivated for her recovery.

These connections that the volunteer team made helped the patients recover. I learned that along the way. People need connection, even when they don't realize it. Without connections or without supportive family or friends, tragic or difficult situations are unmanageable.

A second thing I learned was that in a hospital there is fear. People think, *This injury or illness happened to me, and what if I don't get well? What are all these people talking to me about? What am I supposed to do? What about that medical intervention? What if it doesn't work?* It is scary.

I also got involved with the spiritual care folks. I asked the chaplains many questions about life, grief, and being in the hospital. I was curious about their relationships with patients. Sister Carmen talked to me about spirituality and spiritual care, and I became more involved in my own spiritual connection.

One thing that was very difficult, and which led me to being a hospice volunteer, were the patients who learned they wouldn't be going home or who were readmitted for end-of-life care. That brought back memories of my brother going through this whole thing. Instead of hiding from these triggers, I wanted to face them head-on.

Some of the patients looked at me and pleaded. "I'm scared. I'm going to hospice. Does that mean the end?"

I didn't know how to approach it. How to talk to them. So I decided to go to the hospice training and then became a hospice volunteer. I was still volunteering at the hospital, and it was important to me to have no restrictions on helping, to be able to talk to any patient in need about their feelings. Especially as they were pushing the end of life.

I learned how to do a life review during my training. In the life review, I learned to delve into the deep emotions and memories of the people I was interviewing. The best part of this was the connection to another person to talk about their greatest memories, their most passionate loves, their dreams, and their fears. I enjoyed visiting veterans like me in their homes to learn about their lives when they were facing the end. There was always an immediate bond. There was also a program called We Honor Veterans,[27] where people who served our country were honored by completing pinning ceremonies or flying a flag. I participated in many of these beautiful moments where family members would share their stories and how proud they were. Telling these stories was therapeutic. It was great for grief. I wanted to ensure that anyone sharing their story with me knew I was there, that they weren't alone, and no matter what their experience, we had fought for this country with the same love in our hearts. I was invited to funerals of veterans for whom I'd completed a life review, which was overwhelmingly powerful for me. I was able to share with their family members, and I was able to share the story. I was able to provide that final chapter.

I even did a life review for myself. So much of my life was caring for others. I gave 8,500 hours of my time to volunteerism. I realized that what I had given back was a gift. The time I gave meant something to me, it filled a space for me that was empty with the loss of my brother and mom, but it was also fuel for patients to stay motivated and continue to recover. I saw my impact many years ago when I fell and broke my leg. I had been out of town, and this hospital ensured that I would be transported back here for my treatment. I stayed to do my full rehabilitation.[28] I had nurses, doctors, and even administrators visiting me and rooting for me. I had helped others in this same hospital, and now they were able to support me when I needed it most.

These connections that I had with my community made life interesting and heartwarming. My life was great because of what happened to me. I learned, and I was appreciative of the lessons, the help, and the support. But most of all, I was proud of myself. I was proud of how much I was able to listen and of how many people I'd met who felt supported in their journeys through illness because of my time.

—Gil, community volunteer (San Diego, California)

Some time ago, I took over the care of a patient who had developed an unanticipated, severe toxic infection days after a significant, traumatic injury. No one believed he would survive the first night. His fight through illness with infection rivaled that of a warrior, and the team prayed and pulled for him to come through. We needed a win. We had recently lost a young patient unexpectedly. We were beaten down and de-energized, and we wanted so badly for this patient to survive and thrive.

His story made me think of the *Little Engine that Could.*[29] For those who haven't read the children's story or who need a refresher: The engine wants to help a passenger train up the mountain, but she is considered too small and inexperienced to do so. The engine is the only one who believes she can accomplish the mission. For patients who are going through a challenge with survival, for teams who may be experiencing burnout or are trying to meet an unattainable goal, and for families who are praying bedside day and night, their resiliency becomes the fuel for the medical engine.

Where does the resiliency of humanity come from? The little engine believed in herself, but there wasn't a tremendous amount of support to push the other train up the mountain, was there? As I went back through the story, I saw it differently. The passenger train needed an engine to get it up the incline. The little engine saw an opportunity to help and was willing to put her all into the effort. Maybe the other trains were warning the engine of the odds, barriers, and burdens of going uphill. They were experienced. They had been up the mountain before, some many times. They knew the struggles that the little engine would have. The toys on board the passenger train believed that the little engine could help, and they rooted her on. This was a story of one little engine who found her personal motivation amplified by the power of those around her. She believed in herself and in the cause, got up the mountain, and had everyone cheering her on in the end. There were many parallels to my patients and to my own experiences while building the Generational Health program and providing care for ill and injured patients.

—Diane Wintz (San Diego, California)

Part Three

To work as a team, and to achieve a goal for the betterment of someone else's life, that is to have succeeded. Providing more time or more comfort is to have listened, internalized, and addressed the need. In health care, this is how legacy is made: in being the change factor for the outcome. Prioritizing patients adds a positive spin, making the process of health care purposeful and meaningful.

WHEN CHOOSING A DOCTOR for myself, I look for someone who treats me like they would their own family member. I want a physician who actively acknowledges that I have a whole life beyond the moments spent in a hospital or clinic. Hospitalization does not define life. Life is so much bigger than an illness, injury, or surgery.

—Diane Wintz (San Diego, California)

Leaving a Legacy

Legacy is the mark or the impact made. It is the piece of each of us that changes the course of other people's lives. To give of yourself, to impact someone else, to be a force remembered. For your memories to be cherished and stories told to those who come after you, that is to have left a legacy.

I'M A RETIRED SHARP employee. I worked for Sharp Grossmont for forty-two years as an occupational therapist, and now I am coming into my second year of retirement. It was hard to step away from health care because I loved making a difference, and I loved working. I am proud of that part of my story; of how many people I supported through recovery and rehabilitation. It meant something to me to bring hope and resiliency to my patients. I always prioritized the patient ahead of their illness or injury. I didn't treat strokes; I treated people who had strokes. I reminded myself with each intake that I had treated thousands of people with a stroke, but this was the first time this person in front of me had ever had a health problem, and now he had a stroke, and he had never experienced this before. For this person, this was a personal experience that deserved my respect and my time. This person needed to know that with my expertise and his motivation, he would see improvement in his function. It was critical for me to know him—what mattered to him, what was meaningful. What did he want to be able to do that he couldn't do now? How could I help him get back to that baseline?

I taught my children and my grandchildren to find occupations that they loved so that they would never mind getting up and going to work in the morning. I used to wake up feeling anxious and excited to go to work, to meet new people and to figure out how I was going to help. I couldn't necessarily change the big picture, but I could make a difference. When I retired, I felt lost. I'd lost the immediate ability to help, but I still wanted to positively impact people; otherwise, why was I on this planet?

I'm now making a difference by volunteering. I work with people as they are passing away through the 11th Hour program,[30] and I am also a cuddler in the NICU. These things have helped me stay connected. I think about this dichotomy of caring for patients at end-of-life versus cuddling in the NICU. Both populations are vulnerable and receptive to care. The perspective is invaluable. I feel like I am making a connection in a different but critical way.

In both the NICU and the 11th Hour program, there is a person who appreciates my time but who cannot tell their story. From the little bit of information I may be given from the family or from nurses, I try to know them in whatever way I can. That connection is reinforced when I get a weak squeeze in my hand as I am leaving the bedside, or through the comfortable scrunch and cry from the newborn. My time with them may be finished, but they felt me there, and they let me know.

I was reflecting on Generational Health. I'd never heard of that term during my forty-two active years, but it makes sense that it focuses on every age and stage of development, and the needs that go along with those stages. I look at my own life and how things have changed. I realize that if I were to be hospitalized, there could be changes in my body, my function, or my cognition. And if someone were caring for me, I hope they would be sensitive that this may be a new world for me.

—Darlene, retired occupational therapist (San Diego, California)

I hold a special place in my heart for the older adult population, particularly those with dementia. In my early teens, I grappled with attempting to make sense of how my paternal grandmother, a Holocaust[31] survivor, had gone from living a vibrant postwar life—sharing her empowering story of survival with anyone and everyone—to not recognizing her loved ones' faces when my family and I flew across the country to visit her in Florida. My Grandma Marysia's favorite song was "God Bless America";[32] I have a profound memory of her singing it with pride in her bed at the memory care center where I last saw her. In 2007, she died from complications related to Alzheimer's disease. We sang her favorite song at her funeral to honor her influential legacy of resilience—moving from Poland to America after experiencing the unthinkable horrors of the Holocaust. The loving memories I had with my grandmother were incredibly meaningful. Little did I know that I would develop a deep interest in neuroscience and a true passion for caring for those with dementia throughout my nursing career. Over the years, I gained knowledge and skills and was able to apply them when my mother's father, Grandpa Gigi, was diagnosed with Lewy body dementia[33] at age eighty-four.

My mom was frantic when she called me. Gigi had fallen in the middle of the night and was enroute to the hospital. I was about to start graduate school, and being the only member of my family with medical training, I felt compelled to drive to Los Angeles to see Gigi with my own eyes. When I saw him in the hospital, he was frail and delirious and was not cracking his usual clever jokes. My family did not know all the questions they needed to ask or how to navigate the next steps. I assessed him, spoke to his nurse to find out what work-up had been done, and helped coordinate his discharge plan with the case manager.

I settled him at home and stayed the night to make sure he was safe as my grandmother wasn't able to set up a caregiver until the following day. I answered the home health nurse's questions that my family couldn't. My knowledge and experience proved to be vital in addressing Gigi's needs and ultimately made it possible to facilitate a smooth transition out of the hospital. At the end of my visit, Gigi asked me, "Have you ever thought of becoming a nurse? You'd make a great one." When his sense of humor returned, I knew he was on the mend. His witty banter managed to hide the severity of his dementia. Unfortunately, Gigi was hospitalized again after a fall in January of 2021. We were unable to visit him in the hospital due to visitation restrictions. He had not seen a familiar face for three weeks and developed severe delirium.

As challenging as the decision was, we transitioned him to a hospice home where we were able to say our goodbyes before he passed. I wrote a eulogy—my euloGigi as I called it—and read it during his memorial service via Zoom as it was during the height of the COVID-19 pandemic.

My EuloGigi

When I think of Gigi, I think of a man larger than life; a man of class, full of authentic charm. A kid at heart and one of the happiest, healthiest, and most humorous of humble human beings that I will ever know. Gigi taught me many life lessons. His attitude of gratitude reminded me to be grateful for the little things in life. He taught me to be a good human. Make smart decisions and care sincerely for others. But also, above all, to prioritize my own happiness—he would often call just to ask if I was happy. He showed up for me in so many ways and continues to give meaning to my life even now that he's gone. He taught me how to play tennis and attended as many of my games in high school as he could to cheer me on and, of course, correct my form. I am still in awe of how he was an ambidextrous ping-pong player. What a cool grandpa I had! He also taught me how to swim. I got my love of chocolate and dark turkey meat from him—I'd always save a drumstick for Gigi at Thanksgiving.

Can anyone guess his drink of choice? Yes, you probably knew without hesitation that it was an Arnold Palmer. He always carried Eclipse gum, Altoids, and a nail file everywhere he went—in his office drawer and glove compartment, even in his man purse. He was so fresh, classy, and clean on every occasion. Each article of his tasteful clothing and his size-twelve shoes were always perfectly organized and maintained in mint condition. Gigi had a voice like Sinatra, loved to perform, and created a few songs of his own. There was a song dedicated to his older sister Horty, called "My Sweet Hortence," and then … there was a song about "The Flu Bug" which, with no surprise, he sang to the emergency room physician last year after he fell. The doctor was wondering why he was in such good spirits.

Having three daughters and seven granddaughters, he felt compelled to protect all of us, including Mimi, his one true love. He was the ultimate everything. The ultimate family guy being his favorite role, he was our go-to guy for life advice. When I came out to him a few years ago, he said, "I am not going to try and change you, I just want you to be happy."

The last time I saw him in September, when he still had his wits about him, he met my girlfriend Sarah. He told her he was a hit man in Chicago—she thought he was serious. A while later, he called to ask how my "lady friend Monica" was doing. I couldn't tell if he was joking about forgetting her name. Turns out, he was really good at covering up his dementia with his sense of humor, so we didn't realize how long he was declining. Nevertheless, the simple act of him acknowledging my authentic self was validating.

Wow. I just love the kind and considerate human he was. Gigi had no regrets about life. He taught me to believe that all people are worthy of respect. No matter the differences, everyone had a place on this earth. Gigi would never tolerate treating someone unkindly. He stood up for the underdogs. He lived life with purpose and inspired others to do the same. Everyone who knew Gigi respected him for his wit and clever character. He had no fears about what people would think of him. He could walk into a room, and he would gravitate toward anyone without hesitation. He had an affinity to talk to literally everyone and anyone. Strangers? Your high school crush? Babies? Any living thing, he'd talk and form a connection. He'd make everyone feel welcome and comfortable with his warm, engaging conversations. You could call it the gift of gab. He had this thing about him where he could connect on some level with anyone. With his sunny disposition, you could look into his eyes and feel at ease by his presence alone. It was no wonder everyone wanted to sit next to Gigi at the dinner table, or at a baseball game or school event. Just being around him … you knew it was going to be a good time. When he meant business, though, there would be no question. He commanded respect, and no one would ever think twice about undermining his wisdom. He knew when to laugh and when to be serious. He knew how to brighten your day, brighten up a room.

Anyone who knew Gigi knew his clever sense of humor. Mimi probably heard his same jokes at least one hundred times … you would know it by her soft giggle or her eye roll. Even close to the end, I would just be in awe of his wit. Only a few months ago, I brought my dog Penny over to see him, and she was rolling around on the floor. Gigi said, "Penny, you won't grow up to become a nickel if you keep that up!" He had a knack for witty comebacks. I will miss his annual calls on my half birthday where he would sing every other word of the happy birthday song to me. Not only would he call just to make sure I was happy, but he would also often call just to tell me he loved me. Sometimes, I would let my phone go to voicemail just so I could remember his voice. I will cherish the voicemails I have saved forever.

I know he loved all of us so deeply. I know he was proud of me for becoming a nurse … I am pretty sure that was the first thing he would tell people about me, even strangers. Just starting grad school this past fall to become a nurse practitioner, I will continue to make him proud and serve the older adult population with a full heart of compassion in his memory.

I hope he knew how much I cared that we honored his wishes at the end of his life. With comfort and safety being top priorities, his final breath was taken in a home called Sunshine Place—not just a pleasant name, the wonderful staff there allowed us to say our goodbyes, something (given the COVID-19 restrictions) which a lot of families didn't have the opportunity to do. I recognize how lucky we were to have had the opportunity to tell Gigi in his last moments how loved he was by so many. I told him he was my favorite human and how handsome he was. I held his hand and placed my hand on his chest over his heart. I brushed my fingers through his hair and put lip balm on his lips. Everyone knows how highly Gigi valued his appearance. My sister Jaclyn played "Fly Me to the Moon" by Frank Sinatra and squeezed his hand to the beat. My mom told him it was OK to go and that we would all be alright, that we had each other, something I knew he needed to hear. I kissed his forehead, and I told him his legacy would live on forever.

I leave you with this, the quote I read to Gigi at Sunshine Place—the same farewell quote he read at his retirement party when he was seventy-eight years young, a true testament of what Gigi embodied: "To laugh often and much; to win the respect of intelligent people and the affection of children; to earn the appreciation of honest critics and endure the betrayal of false friends; to appreciate beauty; to find the best in others; to leave the world a bit better whether by a healthy child, a garden patch, or a redeemed social condition; to know even one life has breathed easier because you have lived. This is to have succeeded."[34]

I can only hope to leave a legacy as great as Gigi's.

—Ari, Generational Health nurse practitioner (San Diego, California)

My siblings and I worked on construction sites from around the age of twelve. We didn't get paid; it was our family duty. My dad instilled in us a strong sense of responsibility. We were accountable for our actions, with no room for excuses. He set an example in everything he did—how he treated strangers, his work crew, and our family. His strength was in actions, not words. We knew what he valued and how he expected us to behave. His impact was felt even when he wasn't in the room. And when he died, we continued to live up to that expectation and with those virtues. He left a legacy through his hard work and outstanding character. He was honest and selfless. I hope to leave even a fraction of what he did. My goal is to leave people feeling better than they did before they met me, even if it's just for a moment. I may not live up to everything my dad was, but I believe he would be proud of me, and that feeling is invaluable.

One of the greatest opportunities I've had is caring for the aging population. Treating them holistically, completely, and addressing not just a single issue but the whole person, including their spiritual side, has been incredibly fulfilling.

A year or so ago, I visited Charles, one of our cardiac patients, at home. He was facing an upcoming procedure for his heart. When I arrived at the home, his wife greeted me with a huge smile, and I could smell freshly baked cookies. She sat me in the living room, and we began chatting. I was enjoying my time with her so much that I almost forgot that I was there on business. The cardiac team needed a better sense of her husband's functional status, so I was there to assess him in his activities of daily living. She took me to the back of the house where the living quarters were. The long hallway leading to their bedroom was covered in photos: family vacations, holiday parties, moments frozen in time. Charlie was smiling, tan, debonair, and young. I saw snapshots of his life and moments that mattered to him.

I encountered Charlie in bed. He was smaller than I thought he would be—thinner, frail. He needed his wife's assistance to sit up, but once he was sitting with her supporting his back, he reached his hand out and shook mine. His hands were bony and cold, lacking strength. His breathing was labored, as it typically was with heart failure patients. We needed to do a walking trial, so his wife asked me to hold him up while she grabbed his walker. We both supported him, one of us on each side, while he wobbled to a standing position. I then watched him feebly take two steps forward before he indicated for the chair.

I returned to the office to review his records. These showed that he had arrived to his previous appointments by medical transport in a wheelchair. Based on those previous appointments, there was no acknowledgment about how much care his wife was providing. The procedure had been scheduled based on those office appointments without a true view of life at home. Based on what I had seen, he would not tolerate a procedure. He wasn't an appropriate candidate, and he and his wife deserved to hear that from the medical team. The once-rugged, handsome family man who had enjoyed time on the water and time with his friends was now aging in place and nearing the end of his life. They never would have had that opportunity to talk about how the procedure could steal the small bit of independence he had if I hadn't gone to their home. He might have gone forward with the procedure and not recovered. That procedure—and its outcomes—may have prevented him from going home again. All of this—this visit to their home, my assessment, my counseling—all of this was possible and part of the process with Generational Health. Generational Health nurses and physicians were responsible for teaching me and the team about the impact of vulnerability on recovery.

What matters most to patients can differ from their medical needs. While a heart problem can be evaluated myopically, that misses the bigger picture of life and what goals are realistic. For Charlie, sure, having an operation or a procedure would have fixed his heart issue, but he wasn't surgically ready or strong enough to undergo that type of stress. It would have completely knocked him out and down. It took me being in their world and seeing it all to help them both understand that going forward with a surgery or a procedure would be the wrong move. That was the way in which I could support them best, by *not* scheduling him for a procedure; and oddly, it felt great to be in that position and to be trusted to do that.

Most patients don't want their legacy to end with illness, frailty, or being a burden on others. It's a common fear. By providing tools to help patients stay as healthy and independent as possible, we can help them be proud of their entire life, including its final chapter.

—Annette, cardiopulmonary program manager (San Diego, California)

Many years ago, I cared for a young patient who suffered a gunshot wound to the head. He was critically injured and dependent on machines for survival. Based on the injury, he was expected to require machine support forever. Our team continued to care for him until his family disclosed that his wishes would be to stop. Several months after his death, I was called to court to testify as an expert who had provided medical care. During the testimony, it was suggested that the family's decision to terminate life support was the inciting deadly event, not the gunshot wound. I avoided his parents' eyes on me in that court room. I walked to my car with my head down and got out of there as quickly as I could, but I couldn't get the feeling out of my heart. His parents had decided to move forward with organ donation, and that young man saved five other lives with his donation. I went through my days repeating that court moment—the way I felt slammed, like the wind had been knocked out of me. The way I questioned whether I had guided the family in the right direction. How they must have been feeling about the statement from the defense: "Didn't he die because you removed life support?" I couldn't get it out of my head. I couldn't stand thinking about it. And I questioned every case after, even knowing that survival was not going to be possible or that function would never be regained. And then, about eight months later, I received a colorful envelop in the mail. I didn't recognize the return address. The letter inside read as follows in slow, slanting cursive:

Dear doctor,

You deserve my family's immense appreciation for your efforts in trying to save my son. The reality of his situation was tough, but you handled the courtroom and the defense attorney with grace. My son's life carried value to the lives of five recipients of his organs. His double lung transplant went to a twenty-two-year-old man with cystic fibrosis. That beautiful man has become family to us and has comforted us in our grief. He was recently at Thanksgiving dinner sharing all of the amazing things that he has done this year. While I miss my son more than I can say, I am so proud of his final moment, this gift of donation to a complete stranger who is now family. We never questioned your guidance. We made the right choice.

—Anonymous, surgeon (Baltimore, Maryland)

Embracing Life's Final Chapter

To be present at end-of-life, to actively listen, to pose questions, to build memories, and to realize the imminence of death and uncertainty of health and life is to respect and honor the uniqueness of that person's experience. It is a beautiful moment that deserves peace, warmth, and love. As it was when that person entered the world as a newborn, so should it be as we exit life, making the experience as comfortable as possible and creating meaningful memories for those left behind.

WHEN WE LEAVE THIS world, it's the memories of us that truly matter. The memories are cherished and protected by those who loved us. It's about how people remember us and the marks we leave behind. Our contributions and the positive changes we make can create a ripple effect for those who remain.

Everyone views life and legacy through their own unique perspective. Most people want to leave a lasting impression on those they leave behind. They want their family to remember them a certain way and feel that their support and love will continue even after they are gone.

I went through this with my dad. He was my person. I went to him with everything about my life that needed examination, evaluation, judgment, or decision-making. I had very little time to adjust to the idea that I was going to lose him. He was diagnosed with cancer and had a very fast decline. He lost weight and no longer looked like himself, and he was fatigued and couldn't maintain focus on our conversations. We couldn't have kept up our previous pace even if we had wanted to; the disease stole him in front of my eyes.

Hospice created a comfortable experience for him, but what it did for me and the comfort that it gave me was really the inspiration for me maintaining a relationship with hospice and providing that experience for other families. It would have been so easy for me to walk away with the negative memories of him being sick, but instead, they encouraged us to work on memories even while he was alive. Their attention to both of us gave me the strength to get through my dad's death—the event I dreaded the most in life.

In hospice, we understand that those memories are components of the end-of-life journey. Discussing legacy or end-of-life can be delicate, even though this is the stage when hospice often enters. Building rapport is essential for having meaningful conversations about these topics. People need to feel comfortable opening up about this part of life. Often, thoughts about death are private and haven't been openly shared. It's a beautiful moment when people can talk openly about life, peace, death, and legacy. These conversations can bring families together in ways they haven't experienced before, with an honesty and rawness that carries beauty. The journey they take in their final chapter defines how they want to be remembered, and they can shape that legacy.

—Tegan, hospice navigator (San Diego, California)

My dad had a long history of cardiac disease which started in 1981, when I was in fourth grade. He was thirty-six years old, younger than I am now. He underwent five bypasses in one surgery, rendering him weak and unable to father the way he wanted to. The heart problems stole his energy. There were many things he couldn't do with me, but he listened and taught me the importance of family and keeping negativity on the sidelines.

His health was a constant threat to his life, but the way he dealt with that was through denial and avoidance. He would not take part in a what-if conversation. Maybe he thought of it as a burden we would have to bear; so instead, it was not discussed. It actually made me worry more, and that drove an interest to help and support him, to intervene, to get him better. It was what led me to health care. A way to have education and knowledge. It soothed that inner child who was terrified by the unknown. As I became experienced in my chosen field of nursing, I saw subtle and important changes in those around me. My dad's breathing was telling. It was loud, raspy, and gasping—indicative of heart failure. Heart failure that could be supported medically, symptoms that could be quelled with medication management. Unfortunately, he was not the type to admit to symptoms, and my mother supported him even when he was being stubborn.

At this point, I was the expert. I knew that he was not doing well and was not listening.

When I finally told him that he had congestive heart failure, he immediately denied what I knew to be true. I realized that in his denial was a powerful, silent, and deadly inaction which was inadequately tempered against my obsession to get him treated. Because he didn't believe there was an issue, that issue was not being addressed.

In 2010, I got a call from my mom that my dad was in the ED. "The doctor said your dad has severe heart failure."

Obviously.

Only now he didn't have as much of a voice. His strength and energy were down. He couldn't argue with us like he wanted. He succumbed to the medical interventions that we thought were best. His heart was now supported by an implanted defibrillator.

He loved to travel. This was a real joy for him. He could no longer travel alone, but we had an opportunity to travel as a family and see my sister. I was really anticipating this trip and encouraged him to take it. I wanted to bring him this gift of activity and love for life. About two weeks before we were supposed to leave, my dad passed out at the wheel while driving. Somehow, luckily, he was not injured, and he did not hurt anyone.

Everything changed after that, and it would be up to us to make life-impacting decisions for him. He was never going to drive again. We made numerous changes in the home for accessibility. This was a bigger deal than just a car accident. He had lost the ability to safely care for or make decisions for himself. We debated if it was safe for him to take the last trip he would ever take. The car accident had been a major smack in the face to my family members about his general health with heart failure.

He really wanted to go, so we completed the vacation, but he declined during and after. Back at work, I was talking to the cardiac coordinator. She suggested that my dad might benefit from a left ventricular assist device (LVAD) or transplant. He still met the age criteria and had enough reserve to possibly get through the process, which included a big operation and then a lifetime of careful follow-up, cardiac rehabilitation, and appointments. He would need to come to San Diego, though, because these interventions were not being offered near him. We decided as a family to get him listed for possible transplant, and we waited.

The waiting and the unknown were so stressful. If he didn't match a heart transplant donor, he wouldn't survive. If he received a match, would he want it? Would he consent? Would it work? It was agony to wait. And then there was my insider knowledge: If a heart became available to him, it would be because someone else's life had ended. And that was a really hard thing to pray for.

On June 22, 2012, after several weeks of waiting, we got the call that there was a heart available for him. The energy and the breath went out of the room for a minute, and then we were riding a wave. That day is forever etched in my memory.

It was both celebratory and terrifying because he would be going through a very complicated and risky operation. There was also the undertone of sadness and mourning for the family who had lost their loved one. We were eternally grateful to have this organ, this heart, that would give life back to my dad.

The transplant news came on the one day when my mom hadn't come to the hospital. She'd just needed some time to herself, and she'd happened to not be there when the call had come in. I raced home to get her so we could get moving with the next steps.

It was a whirlwind from there with things moving quickly. The surgeons came to the room, talked to us, and rolled him into the OR around 7:30 p.m. I went home to quickly shower, and I planned to come back. I couldn't help with the surgery, and it was going to be a long night. I needed a few minutes of self-care and quiet. I still feel like I have to justify my decision to leave the hospital, even though I know that it is the best for families and it is what is recommended during long hospitalizations of loved ones.

My uncle called me at home. I knew it wasn't going to be good news. I had been home for less than one hour. The doctor was on the phone.

The cardiac surgeon asked me, "What are your dad's wishes? As we started the operation, he had an arrest. What do you want to do?"

I couldn't breathe. "Do everything until I get there."

My mind flashed to my patients. I thought about how often I had been involved in end-of-life conversations for others, and how little I understood the emotions. In that moment, I was on the other side, making decisions for my dad that he never wanted to make for himself. I knew he could not endure a life on machines or with continued heart failure that was progressive. We had already taken every joy away from him months earlier.

Ultimately, we said goodbye to him during the operation. That was the hardest decision we have ever had to make. The hardest decision I've ever had to help my mom make.

My dad would never have made a decision about his end-of-life care, and I think that was part of the legacy. He dealt with chronic illness from the time he was a young man. Putting wishes down in writing … he never did that; we never did that. We were left scrambling. It put things into perspective for me. I was the medical expert in the family, and I had been unsuccessful in getting him to a decision about his care limitations. After we made the decision, we questioned it even though we knew it was the right one given his circumstances.

Today, my mom has an advance health-care directive. We asked her what she wanted while she could still answer for herself. She now has dementia, so we planned well. My mom made all her own arrangements ahead of time. Everything is ready for us; all we have to do is call a number.

—Eddie, critical care services director (San Diego,
California)

When I was fourteen years old, I had my first experience with a family loss. I was a freshman in high school. I remember going to volleyball practice and then coming home to hear my mom speaking to her mother, Grandma Millie, on the phone about my Grandpa Howard.

I was listening in, and I overheard my mom say, "He had a stroke? Oh no, where is he? Woodland Hills? OK, I'll be over there soon."

I said, "Mom, can I go with you?"

She paused, but then said, "Yeah, OK. Let's go."

We drove thirty minutes to the hospital, which felt like forever. When we arrived, we were greeted by my aunt, who was tearful.

She said, "I don't know if you want to see him like this."

I thought, *Like what?* I didn't know what to expect, but I thought I could handle anything. I was an invincible teenager. My strong-willed personality beamed in full force, and I thought I could save the day … but I couldn't.

My grandpa was on life support. It was my first experience seeing someone I loved with a tube in their mouth connected to a ventilator. His eyes were open, but he couldn't talk. This was the same person we'd just spent a long weekend with in Las Vegas a month prior. We'd walked the Strip and gone to Treasure Island; it had been one of my favorite childhood memories. This was the same person who had taught me how to play card games and who always snuck me Werther's butter candies. My grandparents on my father's side had passed away before I was born, so Grandpa Howard was my only grandfather.

When I saw him after his stroke, on machines and without the ability to talk, I was overcome by emotion like a tidal wave. It hit me so fast, I ran out of the room, completely unprepared. I was so mad at myself for not being able to handle this.

I told my mom, "I'm so sorry … I want to go back in."

When I went back in, I had a feeling it may be the last time I would see him. I told him how much I loved him. I thought he tried to mouth it back, but the tube was preventing him from doing so. That was devastating, but I knew how he felt, even if the words couldn't be said.

That evening, the family decided to shift to comfort. Only my mother was at the bedside when he took his last breath, and she questioned if she had been chosen to experience that vulnerable moment. She felt the sassafras of emotions: happy and sad, cursed and blessed at the same time. Listening to my mother navigate her experience, and reviewing my own experience, contributed to how I help others now, although I said at the time that I never wanted to step foot in another hospital again. I was terrified but also determined—a horrific blend of vulnerability, sadness, desperation, hope for something better, and peace—a normal, human response to the loss of someone so special. I will always attribute blackjack and butter candies to him. This was my first generational loss.

Fast-forward a decade and a half, and Grandma Millie, who had been grieving the loss of Grandpa Howard, was living an active life surrounded by supportive family and friends. She began developing early signs of dementia in her mid-nineties. She was the matriarch of the family. She and Grandpa Howard hosted every single holiday at their home, the same home in which their five children had grown up. My earliest memories of that house were of me crawling on top of an antique three-foot-tall treasure box my grandmother used for blanket storage in the living room. My siblings and cousins would play hide and seek, memorizing every nook and cranny. Neighbors were strangers who quickly became family. These neighbors in my grandma's later years became essential to her caregiving circle.

Soon after Grandma Millie turned ninety-seven, she was hospitalized with a serious infection: sepsis. With her underlying moderate dementia, we quickly learned the hospital was not a favorable place. She underwent surgery to fix a blockage of her bile duct, but overnight, her condition was very unstable. She developed delirium and was not herself. This was the matriarch of our family, the glue that kept us together, the woman who hosted all our holiday gatherings, who raised five children, and always made her opinion known—a fearless, driven, compassionate woman who did not back down to anything. She was innately stubborn but incredibly gracious and giving. She taught me and the other women in our family to be independent, driven, and strong. When her illness brought her to the hospital, she made it clear even with moderate confusion that the hospital was no place to be kept. She was adamant about going back home. She was adamant that she would eat food, even if it meant a complication. She was adamant that she would be released, even if it meant hiring 24-7 caregivers to keep her safe and secure. A stranger hired for the 24-7 care became a key companion for the rest of her days at home. Neighbors were family, caregivers were family, and family was, of course, family until she took her last breath in her home at the age of ninety-nine. Some of my family members were disappointed she didn't make it to her one hundredth birthday, but I reminded them, "She was on her one hundredth year ... we start at zero." No amount of time felt like enough at the end.

No amount of grief prepared me for the next tragedy of our family, the loss of my Uncle George. Uncle George, or Gruncle as I affectionately named him, provided respite for my parents by moving my sister, brother, and me into his home between my fifth and sixth birthdays. This was necessary as my mom sought answers to stabilize her health and my dad pulled all-night shifts while working for the Los Angeles Police Department (LAPD). With Gruncle we lived a more rural lifestyle filled with sports, hobbies, adventures, and good company. Gruncle was the kindest soul with a heart of gold, but he was also strict, which made it feel more like home. Living with him gave us an opportunity to know him and to get close to him. He always gave an open ear, listened to our stories, and offered the best advice. He was the head landscaper for the university for decades, but a few years ago, his hand developed a tremor while he was doing the thing he loved most. His Parkinson's disease advanced quickly. This was the yin and yang—a curveball without reason—that something he loved so much would uncover a disease that would take his life. This incredible person who had compassion for everyone was now experiencing a terrible, debilitating disease that was affecting everything that mattered to him. He was an adventurous, travel-loving man with a wife who matched his energy and kids who craved his advice as they transitioned to parenthood themselves. Our kids called their great great-uncle Gruncle, too, not only for the generational context but because he was simply beyond great. His journey was cut too short for us all. His decline happened so fast, and I always felt like I could have done more to allay his pain and suffering. I still feel that way, but I also know that it hurts that much because of how much he was loved.

That is the sassafras of life: that so many who are loved can be lost. Existence is so meaningful despite the fragility of it. And yet, the impact of my family at these pivotal moments of my life was undeniable. I ran out of Grandpa Howard's room ready to give up on my dream of nursing because seeing him with a breathing tube was overwhelming and devastating. Seeing the sudden loss of his independence and of his ability to talk was crushing. It took my breath away, and I felt help-less seeing him like that. Grandma Millie bossed everyone into letting her return to her home, and it felt like the right decision to maintain her dignity and her comfort for as long as possible. The hospital was supposed to heal, and this was my first experience where it hadn't done that. The lesson was valuable later when I was caring for others. My Uncle George was a safe refuge for my siblings and me; and later, he was a confidant and a role model for me and my children. I took gifts from these relationships. I learned, and I taught my children the lessons of love, family, dignity, free will, compassion, caring, and friendship.

—Kelly Wright (San Diego, California)

A major part of my day involves talking to patients about end-of-life care and ways to make the process more comfortable or understand their options. While it may seem reasonable to talk about those things when facing a terminal illness or when death is imminent, for most people, the process of dying would go better if there was a plan. On a recent podcast, Kelly and I discussed that death planning is akin to planning a trip.[35] If you are going to travel, you have a destination in mind, arrange lodging, pack a bag, organize your activities, and have definitive preparation to make the most of your time. Why would end-of-life planning be any different than preserving and making the most of the time you have left?

There are benefits to planning. While the timing and mechanism of death often remain unknown until the end, there are many pieces that are common in every situation. For example, how aggressive you would want a medical team to be with your care. Whether you would want to die at a hospital or would prefer to be in your own home, and how to make that happen. The decisions for resuscitation or code status are similar to the original childhood dilemma of choosing based on color or flavor; only this time, the decisions surround quality and quantity of life and what is most important to the individual.

Since the wording of an advance care directive can be vague, most patients are unprepared and lack a comprehensive plan for critical life transitions. When patients are hospitalized with a significant illness or injury, they are often not in a vegetative state and are not immediately terminal, so their advance care directive may be irrelevant to their current situation. If you have never discussed options about what you would want if you were never going to return to a fully functional state, you should discuss it with your loved ones immediately. I hear so often, "My mom never wanted to talk about it." This leaves the adult child, next of kin, or the best friend wondering what the right decision is and struggling with guilt over doing the wrong thing.

A 2022 National Institutes of Health (NIH) study found that over 70 percent of patients preferred to die at home; but in 2017, less than one-third of patients had that opportunity.[36] This suggests that many people do not understand how to achieve a homebound discharge when severely ill or injured or how to make dying at home a reality.

Often, families are unprepared to meet the ongoing health needs of someone who is incapacitated, or they lack a home environment suitable for a newly ill or injured person. The care team may continue to offer aggressive interventions that lead to more hospital time but not necessarily to a more durable recovery while waiting for the family to put limitations on these actions. Families may not realize that their responsibility is to act as a spokesperson for that loved one who cannot speak for themself.

Susan was eighty-one years old when she was involved in a major car accident that rendered her injured and hospitalized. She was with her best friend, Cindy, who had been driving. Cindy and Susan had known each other since they were nineteen years old, and they were best friends. Neither of them had children, and they both had lost spouses along the way. Both women had been injured in the car accident, and they had been hospitalized at different facilities. For the first time in their lives, they couldn't support each other. Cindy was in and out of the operating room, and Susan was on a ventilator in the ICU. Cindy was Susan's power of attorney, but because she was so sick herself, she couldn't speak on Susan's behalf. Susan was severely injured, and critical decisions regarding machine-driven support needed to be made. Cindy, also significantly injured, was frequently in the operating room and unable to participate in the care plan due to her own injuries. Although Susan had some written wishes, the details were vague. She had an advance health-care directive with two alternate health-care agents designated, but both agents were unwilling to make decisions when contacted. This left Susan without a designated decision-maker, risking decisions being made against her wishes.

I was Susan's physician in those critical first weeks. I wanted to do what I believed was best for her quality and quantity of life. She was intubated, had a breathing tube placed, and was attached to a ventilator because she could not adequately breathe on her own. As the days went on, she became weaker. She was on a very low amount of sedative, mostly for comfort with the breathing tube that was going down her throat. She lost muscle and couldn't raise her arms off the bed. She wasn't able to participate in physical therapy at all. Nurses were turning her in bed every two hours to offload pressure points on her back so that she wouldn't get a skin ulcer. It was hard to watch.

I was obligated to continue this level of care because I had no idea what her wishes were for herself. She wouldn't be able to maintain the work required for breathing over time, she wouldn't be able to cough or clear her airway of secretions, and she would be at risk for death from respiratory distress if I removed her from the ventilator. I also couldn't move forward with a tracheostomy (placing the airway in her neck) because this was a procedure that would require consent, which she couldn't provide, and there wasn't a designated decision-maker identified. I was eventually able to get in touch with an attorney who had met with her when she'd originally filed her health-care directives. He had some personal knowledge of her intentions when she'd completed the forms, but he didn't feel comfortable to make her medical decisions, specifically to decide if we should compassionately remove the breathing tube and allow death to occur or if we should push forward with the tracheostomy and place her in long-term care, likely forever, still without anyone identified to make decisions for her later. I called everyone listed on her paperwork, but none of them were willing to decide for her.

This whole time, Susan was the one suffering. Because she couldn't express herself and there was no one to speak for her, she was languishing in an ICU bed, in limbo, with no decisions being made for her care or her long-term management. What really bothered me about this situation was that she probably thought she had made adequate plans for herself. She had a trust and estate planning completed. She had completed these documents with an attorney who had filed them for her. The hospital had copies of these. She had an advance directive that indicated to stop medical interventions if she were brain-dead or vegetative. She'd chosen two women who were the adult daughters of her acquaintances to make decisions for her if her primary power of attorney could not. When I called each of them, they both said the same thing: "We didn't really know her that well." The other problem was that the advance directive was too broad. I couldn't use it outside of those parameters, and she didn't meet them. I was stuck waiting until her attorney finally agreed—as no one had stepped forward, he would work with me to determine the next steps based on my expertise and guidance. We decided together to remove the breathing tube and allow Susan to pass comfortably and naturally.

I walked away from her room thinking about how important it was to understand my loved ones' wishes, the weight of responsibility of being an advocate in a time when my loved ones couldn't speak for themselves, this dire limbo Susan had been in, and this imprisoned medical quandary. I thought of how important it was to get the wishes in writing; but clearly, Susan did have documentation, and it still wasn't enough. I thought about how few people probably realize this shortcoming and how many more times I might find myself in this same boat with someone else. Especially now as the baby boomer generation is aging, and the adult children who are my age are dealing with their aging parents as well as their own children, they are juggling the responsibility toward a generation that is dying and a generation that is just getting started. I thought about how many people my age are probably named as next of kin on someone's advance directive, and how many of them really know and can articulate what that person wants. There is likely little understanding of the impact of long-term care and choices they might make for their parents.

I had to mature into this idea of looking at the big picture when caring for people. A surgical problem equaled a surgical solution, just like an appliance store sold washing machines, not shoes. It was more complicated, though, to take care of people. My patients never knew my stories, and they likely weren't aware of the other team members' biases, ethics, morals, or perspectives, or how these played into life-and-death discussions or decisions. They relied on me to give options, but besides medical expertise, I had experience. I knew that life was bigger than a hospitalization, an illness, or an injury. That options needed to be given with consideration of whether that person could resume life as it had been before. Sassafras—that paradox of experience versus knowledge and judgment—was a necessary component of expertise that came together to result in comprehensive care. This became my obsession, my driving force, and the foundation of Generational Health.

—Diane Wintz (San Diego, California)

Jenny's husband had stage four cancer. It had progressed despite thorough adherence to chemotherapy and radiation. Surgery had been completed. Life was going one day at a time for them. He was able to participate in home rehabilitation where the therapists came to him. Jenny was trying to enjoy life as it was. The last time they were in the hospital was a few months ago. Jenny was a bit frustrated when the doctors again asked about his end-of-life wishes. *Wasn't that written down or available in the chart? Why was it like Groundhog Day with this conversation? Weren't the doctors talking to each other?* One day, he unexpectedly woke up not feeling well, and he knew. Jenny wanted to call an ambulance. She wanted him to be transferred to the hospital where he could be supported. He put his hand on hers and said, "Not this time, Jenny." She looked at him, and his eyes told her. He had an advance care directive, he had a POLST form, they had discussed his wishes many times, and he had her. He was going to approach his end-of-life plan exactly as they had planned together: at home, quietly, in a moment full of love and appreciation.

—Jenny, community member (Encinitas, California)

During the COVID-19 pandemic, patient volume overwhelmed our resources. There was a constant need for doctors, nurses, assistants, techs, therapists, servers, cleaners … you name it. I vividly remember walking down the ICU halls which were filled with IV pumps, drips, nurses in powered air-purifying respirators (PAPRs), and doctors intubating or placing lines and talking on the phones to families. There were upward of double-digit deaths per day, and my job was to palliate the suffering. I would spend countless hours trying to connect patients with their loved ones so I could know the person in the hospital bed. Words would never do justice to the decisions that had to be made during that time. There was a patient who told the health-care team up-front that he didn't want a breathing tube or to be put on a ventilator. He explained, "I lived a good life. If this is the end, then so be it. I want to at least be able to say goodbye with my own voice to my family before I go." His words were raspy and gasping, coming out slow but forceful. I knew he wouldn't survive the night without a machine to support him. I spent the evening at his bedside in an N95 mask and draped from head to toe, making sure I heard him correctly with his sputtering speech, patiently waiting for him to get his words out clearly, making sure I didn't miss any detail about him, his life, and his end-of-life wishes. I connected him with his family, ensured he was comfortable, and allowed him the privacy of a final conversation with his loved ones … on his phone, in accordance with the no-visitors policy.

I was twenty weeks pregnant, and I thought to myself, *I hope this is the right thing.* I was exposing myself to a virus that no one knew anything about. Was I risking my health and the health of my baby to support this man in the last moments of his life? I knew there was risk, but I couldn't turn my back on someone in need of all of the things I had trained to do.

That same moment, Leah was clocking in to her shift. She was assigned to the unit where I was already deep into the day. She and I passed each other in the hall, both of our faces marked with mask creases and fine lines when we smiled for our introduction. She was an extender nurse in the ICU for the pandemic, meaning she picked up extra shifts, coming from the labor and delivery unit. She wanted to be one of the "all hands on deck."

I remember thinking how incredible it was for a labor and delivery nurse to volunteer her time on an ICU shift. She just looked at me and said, "Yes, the units are different in a way, but also it's not that different from taking care of moms and babies. This is the circle of life."

She was right, of course. She was caring for those at the beginning of life, and I was caring for those at the end. We made a great team for families experiencing the generational effects of the pandemic.

She and I became close during our long days and nights. One night, she confided in me. "My husband was a patient here, right here in this ICU. He had an unexpected critical issue and ended up on advanced life support. I knew he wasn't going to do well. I knew he wasn't going to make it. It all happened so fast. He was fine. We were living a beautiful life with our children, traveling every year, and then this thing happened. Being a nurse, it was a nightmare. I knew too much … way too much. I knew his prognosis was terrible, and that he wasn't going to survive. I knew what he would want because we'd talked about it. You know, being a nurse, that's what we do, right? Years ago, in this ICU, I had to make the hardest decision I've ever had to make."

She went on to describe how she was torn apart thinking about her children growing up without their father. "He always told me if he couldn't be a father to our kids, then he wouldn't want to live. I had to ask the team, who was so gracious, so kind, so supportive, and who wanted to fight for him … I had to ask them to stop. That was years ago, and I couldn't step foot in an ICU until COVID-19 hit. I knew I had to help."

My heart squeezed. I could feel this pain like it was my own. I responded with admiration for her courage to make difficult decisions on his behalf and do what she knew was best.

Over the next few months, we were so busy with work that we would see each other in passing, but our time was spent caring for patients and debriefing with our staff. My pregnancy was progressing, but I was so focused on everyone else that I barely even realized I was approaching thirty-eight weeks. My doctor ordered me to take leave. She was worried about my blood pressure and told me to get to the hospital for monitoring. I was rushed to the labor and delivery unit for check-in, was admitted, and was being helped into a gown when I realized Leah was poking her head in at the door. She hadn't forgotten about me! She had promised me all those weeks ago that she would hold my hand for my first delivery.

"Looks like we'll be having a baby soon. Your doctor called from the office letting us know you were coming on over. She said to admit you today, and I get to be your nurse!"

I laughed out loud and immediately felt at ease during a time of uncertainty. She was a comforting presence in another chaotic environment, and I knew everything was going to be fine—and it was. She was only my nurse for the rest of the day shift, so she gave me a huge hug, we took a picture to commemorate the exciting pre-baby moment, and she reported off to the night nurse and then went on her way. The night was full of events with my baby being born early in the morning.

Fast-forward a couple of years, and I had barely seen Leah. We were back to our previous roles: no longer covering the ICU, no longer meeting emergently in labor and delivery. Life took us back to our previous paths. I was on a work call in my office, listening while one of my palliative care colleagues talked about an incredible nurse who was battling terminal illness with poor prognosis and had decided to go home on hospice but wanted to provide gratitude back to her staffing colleagues and invite them to visit on her last day at the hospital.

It was Leah.

My stomach lurched.

The woman who had shared her grief with me and had been there for me during the birth of my son. She was a patient only a couple of floors down. I had to see her. I had to thank her. I had a million things I wanted to tell her.

I didn't want to disturb her, so I was going to turn and leave when she opened her eyes and said in a soft, comforting voice, "Kelly, I'm so glad you are here. Please sit down."

I sat with her. Her voice was kind, but I could tell she was weak.

I said, "I just wanted you to know I'm here."

She responded, "How's Jordan?"

My son. She'd he remembered his name after all this time. I showed her a picture of him at age two. I also went back to the picture of us on the day he was born. "You helped me bring him into this world. I'm so grateful for you!"

She looked at me and smiled. "The circle of life." She continued, "I just never thought my kids would be orphaned at such a young age."

I felt gutted. I felt defeated. I couldn't help. I couldn't save her. I couldn't give the appreciation I felt to her or her children. "Your children will always know what incredible parents they had, what an incredible mom you are. I am here for you and them."

Our eyes filled with tears as we talked for a few more minutes, mostly making sure she had everything she needed at home. We hugged our final goodbye, and I thought to myself, *The circle of life isn't long enough—it has too small of a diameter for those who shine brightly and bestow their light on others.*

—Kelly Wright (San Diego, California)

Lessons Learned

Experience is a gift to give to those who have none. This is especially true in health and in life, where often there is an innate need for human connection, advocacy, a helping hand, a kind word, and support in new and unchartered waters of health, grief, and building strength to face the challenges ahead.

JANE AND HER HUSBAND Bob had a routine. He would get up at 5:00 a.m., throw on a pot of coffee, hop in the shower, and turn on the news. Around 6:30 a.m., he would wander back into the bedroom, rub his wife's back until she gently woke up, and help her to sit up and take her morning medications. The walker would be waiting next to the nightstand. With one arm under hers, he would hoist her into a standing position. Sometimes she needed a little extra massage, especially to her calves, before she could stand. She communicated quietly with a smile or one or two whispered words to show her appreciation. They would make their way to the breakfast nook where they would share a cup of coffee.

They did this every morning for seven years until Jane had an unexpected fall that brought her to the ED where she was admitted. What they didn't realize was that they had fallen into a critical routine for Jane. She needed her medications administered at the exact same time every day, and she needed the established patterns to help her stay oriented. Without those, she became paranoid and refused treatment. She became acutely agitated and combative to her nursing team on the second hospital night. She developed suspicion of the care team, and her husband was the only one who could reliably administer her medications. He was able to come to the hospital to provide support. When he walked into the room, you could see her body relax. He spoke to her in a quiet voice, and she reached for his hand and told him that she loved him.

Health-care teams do not always understand the effects of long-term progressive illnesses on caregivers or families. Many patients with neurocognitive disorders have a muscular component that can impact function. They may also be pattern-driven or dependent on a strict timeline for medication administration. These details can be overlooked with standardized protocols that lack consideration of the individual's needs. The Generational Health team prioritizes the home routine in the hospital as essential. Some patients require personalized care plans because they do not respond as expected to standardized treatments designed for more generalized populations. In certain cases, care may be best provided within the home environment due to the patient's reliance on patterns.

I reconsidered Jane's case and wondered if the hospitalization had helped her. Hospitals healed people, and that was their reputation, but there seemed to be times when that simply wasn't true. Delirium and acute confusion—which manifested either quietly with paranoia or distrust, or loudly with agitation and violence—increased complications and led to lengthy hospitalizations with poor outcomes. There were times when hospitalization just wasn't helpful. I didn't really understand how to communicate that to my patients' families. I didn't know how to explain to a nonmedical person that the hospital could be dangerous. It was weird to see it that way, but after Jane's experience, I questioned if I was always doing the best thing for my patients, and whether it was more therapeutic in certain situations for the patient to stay home.

—Donald, nurse (San Diego, California)

My father was an amazing man, a pillar in his community. Most importantly, he was a great father, and he made everyone feel like they were the most important person in the room. He passed away earlier this year from illness. For me, these last few months have been about reflecting and promoting my dad's legacy in a way that would make him proud.

I learned the power of self-care while I was going through end-of-life care with him. In many of the initial moments of his illness, I attended to the bedside with my nurse brain on. I had a really hard time dropping my nursing background and just being present to spend the time with him focused on him and not on his disease. I realized that I used work and my expertise as a way to escape what was happening with my dad. I used it to escape from the scary moments in life—it was a way to disconnect. As my dad aged and approached his own mortality, I had to remind myself to see him for who he was: a person who had goals, interests, and priorities, even when he was sick. In doing that, I was able to empower him again, but more importantly, I was able to enjoy my time with him. He felt valued when I was able to separate his illness from all the things that were most important to him. It was easier for me to focus on what mattered to him once I realized I was wasting our time together by doing the job of a caregiver. That someone could be brought in with this expertise and alleviate me to get out of nurse mode. I was better doing my nursing job for strangers, not for my dad; and once I realized that for myself, I was able to relax and enjoy the journey, the time we had, and the stories that were buried deep and only came out as the end of his life was approaching. I was able to spend time at the bedside hearing his stories, creating more memories, and learning about him in ways I never had before. I could be part of the family and experience the emotions and camaraderie. I didn't have to be a nurse at the bedside. I could be my dad's daughter, and he could still be dad to his baby girl.

I realized that there were many resources in the community available to both of us. Many were available to me in my bereavement. I didn't have to do any of the journey alone, which was a relief. I leaned on my friends to help me navigate the process. The community lightened the load for me so that I could focus on my dad.

What have I learned from this experience? To lean on others. To tap into resources earlier. To ask friends to join an appointment or take notes. To speak up and be my own advocate. To remind the medical team that I needed to be the daughter and not the nurse/doctor/CEO of the family.

To my fellow nurses: Don't forget to be present. We have a tricky role to balance. In some ways, falling into the role we are used to helps soothe or contextualize the emotions, and maybe that is comfortable when we feel tired or strained. While our knowledge can be a huge benefit to us in utilizing the system, recognizing illnesses, managing medications, and understanding diagnoses, outsourcing the nursing part is key. We don't have to be "on the clock" to be involved. I look back at my own experience, and I know that I used my nursing expertise to hide my fear and apprehension about my dad's illness. But now that he is gone, I realize that sometimes we just have to feel our feelings. (I'm still learning that one.) My dad's greatest lessons came during the hardest part of his life: to care about myself, to acknowledge my emotions, and to accept that it was part of life to be vulnerable.

My dad was a wonderful man who taught me countless lessons in life and now in death. I am proud to be sharing our story, and I'll end with what he wrote me in a letter a long time ago that I just had tattooed on my arm: "Remember that it is OK. Love, Dad."

—Stef, emergency department nurse (San Diego, California)

I was a nursing assistant on the oncology unit when I met Jack, a patient who would change the course of my career. He was a family man, a rock-solid dad and husband, a coach to his son's baseball team, and an outstanding musician. He was undergoing leukemia management, often spending several weeks, month after month, going from home to hospital to home. His course was long and repetitive, the only variation being the countless interactions with strangers who later became comrades, listeners, and fans. He would read newspapers to stay up to date on world events, he would play his guitar, and his wife would fill our staff room with snacks. When Jack was home, the nurses would miss the guitar music and the friendly banter about who had won the baseball game.

When I was in my twenties, I didn't think about the what-ifs. I cared for other people—some of them young, all of them fighting for life—and I began to realize that I wasn't invincible. Life was fragile, and I learned that lesson through the experience of caring for others. Jack was a human superhero, someone who bounced back numerous times to fill my life with light even though the reality was dark. He was dying.

My inner child had so many questions: Why was Jack getting worse despite treatment? Why was this happening to a wonderful person? Why was he encumbered with building a legacy for his wife who was younger than me? Jack was fighting for his family every single day. Infusion, transfusion, recover, repeat. I was so close to my dad, and I thought about Jack's beautiful children who were too young to understand that disease was robbing their experience.

Jack's quick wit and humor never faltered, but he lost the ability to play his guitar. I remember the day his music died, and part of me went too with that reality hitting me hard and deep.

Jack took his last breath while on comfort measures. He had prepared his family the best he could. Their love never wavered; their care never stopped. What Jack did not prepare for, and what he didn't live to see, was his impact on the team and the hole he left. I believed he knew how much we cared, but I didn't know if he anticipated the weight of his loss on our team.

That experience was what I needed to realize the strength of the human spirit, which contains the motivation factor,[37] that thing that keeps a person moving during the toughest parts of life, that resiliency that is demonstrated while dredging through illness or injury. The human spirit is one that wants to live. It wants to fight even in adversity. Living is a gift, and it is mine to enjoy, savor, and experience. I took my love for bedside care and went back to school so that I could support others like Jack in their most difficult moments. I was promoted stepwise to my current position of manager, overseeing the Advanced Illness Management team and Generational Health.

Caring for those who lived full and beautiful lives, who were willing to share their learned knowledge and wisdom, and who benefited from expert care fit perfectly. I learned to be a novice again in certain aspects of management, to be vulnerable, to take more risks, and to lean on my advisers to foster growth, professionalism, beneficence, and empowerment. I learned we should always be operating at our best, shooting for the seemingly intangible, engaging in partnerships and philanthropic opportunities, and advocating for national and international collaborations.

—Kelly Wright (San Diego, California)

My dad had a tremendous influence on me. As a child, I was sort of afraid of him. He had a loud voice and was strict. His moral and ethical compass was impeccable. He had the highest level of integrity and honesty, so I always knew how he felt about me and my actions, which was more appreciated as I got older. He was focused and eidetic, brilliant and curious for facts. We were very close and had many conversations about life and death.

Several years ago, he fell. And because he was on aspirin and Plavix, he wanted to be evaluated for potential injury. He drove himself to the ED that morning and walked a mile from the parking lot to the triage area.

He was found to have a mild traumatic brain injury which did not require surgery. He was admitted for monitoring. I talked to his admitting physician on the phone and agreed with the plan. The admission process took the entire day, so by the time he got to his hospital room, it was late, and the staff moved him from the ED gurney to the bed. The following morning, the physical therapist assessed him, and he needed maximum assistance to sit at the edge of the bed. This led to three extra days of recovery in the hospital for him to regain the strength he had lost in a single day, which had been completely preventable. He had walked into the hospital! Similarly to studies showing that one day of bed rest was equivalent to three days of recovery in older patients,[38] his strength had been lost that quickly.

I learned from him and this experience. Had he been encouraged to be out of bed while he waited in the ED, he would have maintained his strength, and that extra hospitalization would have been avoided. So I brought that story back to the team, and we designed a process to get patients up to a chair in the ED. Seeing someone up and out of bed was an immediate visual change and reinterpretation. When somebody was in bed, covered to the chin with blankets, they looked helpless. I had been guilty of assuming that a person couldn't walk or couldn't care for themselves when I hadn't evaluated their physical function or strength. This assumption had downstream effects such as keeping patients in bed longer than necessary or initiating placement outside of the home without a full functional evaluation.

One way I was able to leave my durable impact was through the construction of the Generational Health program. It was perfect for me and aligned with my field of expertise. This program provided jobs, promotions, experience, and health care-directed, purposeful interaction with the community.

Generational Health was built on experience. Unlike many programs that started with administrative goals, ours began with a single patient's experience. We aimed to improve a better experience for every patient after him. For me, community is what builds programs, sustains motivation, and identifies the need. We care for people as if they are family, and these stories show the insurmountable impact community and family have on the way we care for and interact with others.

It has been incredible to watch people develop the program while doing things they love within their work lives and really making an impact on the care that we provide.

—Diane Wintz (San Diego, California)

I thought about that little girl who played every sport and then decided to be a nurse. In playing sports, I learned about fair judgment, decision-making, reflexes, instinct, disappointment, and achievement. Referees were put on the field to level the game and make the play calls without bias. Their decisions were final, and arguing with them would result in a time-out on a bench. It would shorten playing time. It could lead to a penalty.

Life is so similar.

Jack, Leah, and members of my own family whom I have lost during their health-care journeys—each story holds value and meaning with a learning opportunity, an anchor when I am feeling down, or something to give to a friend at a low point. I keep them close at all times, reflecting back to the moments of care and to their lives as I knew them. I don't think there is any other career where there is constant learning, this level of emotion, or immense fulfillment.

Health-care teams work to win, but they understand that loss doesn't mean failure. Certain days are doubleheaders. Being aggressive has its place; the last seconds of a game can determine the win. In end-of-life care, there are more referees, more play calls, more time-outs, and more buzzers. Questions sometimes don't have answers. There are more concessions. I know that every play holds a lesson, an emotion, and a meaning to the players and to the fans. That there is camaraderie in the moment, the recall, and the replay, with that emotion holding a special place in the memory of that game. There is an appreciation of those childhood lessons, that sassafras polarity guiding the most critical moments of my life—what I give to others and what I take away.

—Kelly Wright (San Diego, California)

Conclusion

Sassafras.
A versatile plant, both healing and harmful. A sacred tool in the hands of the those who value wisdom from the generations before them.

MY PROVISION OF HEALTH care was a personal experience, one that held emotion and meaning. One that led to teaching, building, improvement, and reflection. It was human connection at its finest, the cutting edge of humanity. I was thinking about whole-person care, the essence of Generational Health, and the concept of putting the patient at the center of the health plan. It made sense in a way that was obvious, while simultaneously requiring excessive coordination to do it well. The person going through a health crisis wasn't really at the center; it was more of a circle of support with each participant giving something of themselves in this plan and receiving something back in return. I had never thought about the return—the value received and magnified in this process. How much came from this process. The whole-person care plan needed the provider of the care, the family, the friends or loved ones who made up the "what matters" in that person's life, and the many strangers who floated in and out of the hospital room or the home to give something of themselves. The return was magnified by what each of those individuals took back from that experience—what they taught, built, learned, innovated, and held dear. That was the magic of health. That love and support, the unspoken piece, that part that couldn't exist without human connection.

Thinking back to that candy store, I realize now how meaningful that childhood memory was. That decision to choose an option based on appearance or flavor. Which one really mattered most to me and needed to be considered with the utmost attention? Forty years later, this became the premise of Generational Health, a program based on what was most important to that individual, designed by me and my team, as a reflection of our experience and expertise.

My dad was one of my greatest cheerleaders. He was so proud of me being a doctor. He had heart disease and was often in and out of hospitals, until the last time when there was nothing more that could be done to save him. He could be given more time on earth with machine support, but it wouldn't be quality time. Sassafras has healing powers in small quantities, while in high doses it is harmful. And such is the pendulum of life, when it is clear that life can be salvaged, swinging back to when we know death is coming. I used every experience I had with my dad in some part of the design of Generational Health and how I now care for people. When my dad was hospitalized, I only knew he needed attention. Whether his doctor got to have dinner with his own family that night was not on my mind, even though I was often on the other side of that, skipping family events because someone needed me. After my dad died, I tended to a man who was about his age and needed help deciding on hospice options. That man's family didn't realize the power of my perspective on the counseling I provided. I never share my personal life with patients, but that is what is so special about this book.

On October 29, 2024, we held a Generational Health event with a mission to understand connection through the eyes of our community members. We planned to use that information to continue to evolve our program which focused on older adults. What emerged from the storytelling and short interviews were the voices of our care team. Many of them spoke of personal experiences and the legacy stories of their loved ones that shaped their perspectives in caring for others. Several interviewees gave pivotal examples of family members who had tremendous impacts on their lives.

The Generational Health program was built and grown primarily during the COVID-19 pandemic. I am often asked about how a program was able to get off the ground during a worldwide pandemic, especially one that was so resource-intense. I think a big part of the success was that the staff needed to decompress from tougher cases, to see successes and survival. For me, the program gave me a boost. It was the thing I sunk my time and energy into when I needed a pick-me-up. It was the cure for my burnout, and it fueled my resiliency.[39]

So many of the health-care priorities revolved around quality and quantity of life in the context of a whole person, especially for patients who were facing difficult care decisions or were approaching the end of life. That was the same yin-yang that I experienced as a child when deciding between two reasonable choices, either being relevant based on time of life. Quality is defined by you stating what matters. Quantity is defined by the uncontrollable variable, the thing that remains unknown and unpredictable.

—Diane Wintz (San Diego, California)

I thought about the people I deeply loved and lost, and how many lessons I learned from them, and how precious those moments were. My family clearly made an impact. In reflecting on the stories in this book, I saw that everyone shared how deeply people cared about other people, that there was joy despite heartache, miracles along with tragedy, appreciation for the connection with strangers, and proof that as health-care professionals we would endorse that grief was worth the love and relationship, the experiences and the memories. That resiliency was the manifestation of survival, that we were here for a purpose, and that it was an emotional journey. I considered how often my patients influenced me, and I wondered how often I made a difference for them. I thought about how deep into emotions and the critical portions of life health-care professionals are able to go with their patients, most of whom are strangers before their health-care experience. The pathway is sprinkled with sassafras—the expertise, history, and lessons learned tempered by our own emotional journeys of health care, of caring for others, and of supporting the ill and injured—all while advising, counseling, and guiding patients to make the best decisions for themselves.

Life is fragile, but it is worth the whirlwind of emotions to get to the lessons and to get to the meaning. And it is transcendent to realize how much influence my community has brought to me personally through the legacy stories and the parables that I will carry forward. I thought about the power of one—how much one person can accomplish, how much one person can impact another, how much one person can build—versus the power of community and what a community can affect. Generational Health and my life's work to this point has been to focus on people and what matters most to them in their health or in their lives. This has been my dream realized. I have been the catalyst to spark a movement, with the fuel of human connection nurturing that movement, propelling it forward, and supporting its sustainability. And I feel proud. The stories in this book underscore the value of real people and providers, caregivers who thrive in an environment that fosters the indispensable role of human connection in transforming ideas into reality.

Generational stories are critical to our being. Our patients mirror the most basic part of ourselves, the core of our priorities and the dreams we want to realize.

We chose to be in health care, shaped by our predecessors who knew we could make a difference, one person and one family at a time, by pouring our knowledge, expertise, and most importantly, our generational influence toward those in need. We have shared those stories because what mattered mattered to us.

The experiences shared in this book showcase the tremendous impact people had on our lives. We wanted to emphasize the importance of each chapter of this book—human connection; compassion, dignity, and free will; inescapable truths; what matters matters; advocacy; giving back; leaving a legacy; embracing life's final chapter; and lessons learned—and how each topic was influenced by life events, our stories, our ups and downs ... our sassafras, the powerful plant that was often used as a medicinal tea, serving a therapeutic purpose to the heart of the health-care soul.

—Kelly Wright (San Diego, California)

Thank you so much for keeping us close to your heart and supporting us by reading, remembering, and sharing the stories of all of us. As Bijal (Dr. Patel) said, we love you.

Acknowledgments

WE WOULD LIKE TO thank our colleagues and friends who attended the Generational Health event at the Sharp Prebys Innovation and Education Center in San Diego, California, on October 29, 2024, and who allowed us to reproduce their stories and their interviews to make this book.

We would like to extend immense gratitude to each person who supported Generational Health and the growth of geriatrics at Sharp Memorial Hospital, including the Sachs family for their very generous philanthropic donation to support the program; Bill Littlejohn and Shawna Fallon for their backing of Generational Health; and Tim Smith, Trisha Khaleghi, Chris Howard, and the hundreds of nurses, staff, administrative leaders, and experts with whom we work alongside every day (when we aren't writing).

A heartfelt thank-you also goes out to our families: To Dave, Ashley, Olivia, and Jordan who have encouraged our writing and endured many hours of us reading sections out loud; to our parents who are overwhelmingly proud of our achievements; and in loving memory of Jay who inspired so many of the things we do.

Special appreciation goes to Helene, Jessica, and Ingrid who provided initial edits and guidance on structure and layout and believed in our dream from the very first sentence!

A huge hug and lots of jumping up and down with excitement to Melissa Karren who designed the cover and produced the logo for Jay's Heart.

Finally, to Anna Krusinski, our editor, for taking on this project and providing endless guidance toward perfection, and to Nate Myers for the interior design and layout. Thank you both so much for your time and expertise in helping us complete and publish this novel.

For any reader who is looking for support during a difficult medical illness, injury, or decision-making, you can reach the authors at https://jaysheart.com/.

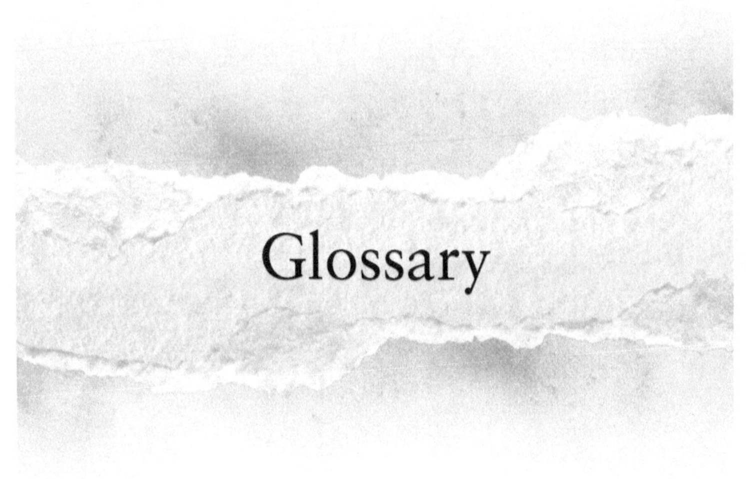

Glossary

Advance health care directive: AHCD

Advanced Illness Management: AIM

Advanced practice registered nurse clinical nursing specialist: APRN-CNS

Center for advanced palliative care: CAPC

Chronic lymphocytic leukemia: CLL

Computed tomography: CT

Do not resuscitate: DNR

Emergency department: ED

Emergency medical services: EMS

Geriatric emergency department accreditation: GEDA

Geriatric surgery verification: GSV

Health volunteers overseas: HVO

Intensive care unit: ICU

In vitro fertilization: IVF

Los Angeles police department: LAPD

Left ventricular assist device: LVAD
Neonatal intensive care unit: NICU
Operating room: OR
Peripherally inserted central catheter: PICC
Physician orders for life-sustaining treatment: POLST
Quick response: QR

Notes

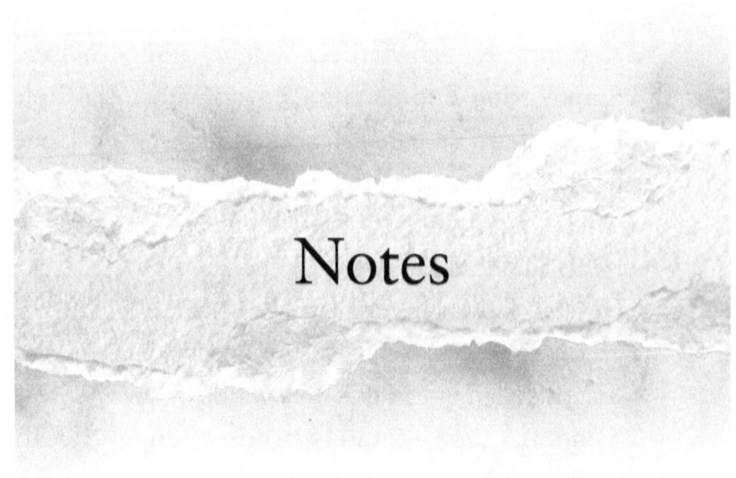

1. Sharp HealthCare, "Generational Health," retrieved August 24, 2025, https://www.sharp.com/services/generational-health.
2. American College of Emergency Physicians, "ACEP Emergency Department," retrieved August 24, 2025, https://www.acep.org/edap.
3. Institute for Healthcare Improvement, "Age-Friendly Health Systems," retrieved August 24, 2025, https://www.ihi.org/partner/initiatives/age-friendly-health-systems.
4. American College of Surgeons, "Accreditation and Verification: Geriatric Surgery Verification," retrieved August 24, 2025, https://www.facs.org/quality-programs/accreditation-and-verification/geriatric-surgery-verification/.

5. D. Wintz, K. Schaffer, K. Wright, and S. Nilsen, "Empowering End-of-Life Conversations: The Role of Specialized Nursing Teams in Facilitating Code Status Changes at Discharge," *Journal of Palliative Care* 40, no. 2 (2024): 176–182, https://doi.org/doi.org/10.1177/08258597241283303.

6. C. Maxwell, M. Dietrich, and R. Miller, "The FRAIL Questionnaire: A Useful Tool for Bedside Screening of Geriatric Trauma Patients," *Journal of Trauma Nursing* 25, no. 4 (2018): 242–247, https://doi.org/DOI: 10.1097/JTN.0000000000000379.

7. Health Volunteers Overseas, retrieved August 24, 2025, https://hvousa.org.

8. S. Parikh, et al., "Chronic Lymphocytic Leukemia in Young (≤ 55 Years) Patients: A Comprehensive Analysis of Prognostic Factors and Outcomes," *Haematologica* 99, no. 1 (2014): 140–147, https://doi.org/ 10.3324/haematol.2013.086066.

9. National Pancreatic Cancer Foundation, "Understanding the Whipple Procedure," retrieved August 24, 2025, https://www.npcf.us/whipple-procedure-pancreatic-cancer-guide/.

10. Sharp HealthCare, "Benefits of Skin to Skin Care: Kangaroo Care Supports Baby Bonding in the NICU," retrieved August 24, 2025, https://www.sharp.com/health-news/kangaroo-care-supports-baby-bonding-in-the-nicu-video.

11. "Ruha," *Wikipedia*, May 25, 2025, https://en.wikipedia.org/wiki/Ruha.

12. "Camino de Santiago," *Wikipedia*, August 24, 2025, https://en.wikipedia.org/wiki/Camino_de_Santiago.

13. Senior Tech Connect, retrieved August 24, 2025, https://seniortechconnect.net/.

14. "Oppenheimer (Film)," *Wikipedia*, August 22, 2025, https://en.wikipedia.org/wiki/Oppenheimer_(film).

15. "Manhattan Project," *Britannica*, retrieved August 24, 2025, https://www.britannica.com/event/Manhattan-Project.

16. D. Kiernan, *The Girls of Atomic City: The Untold Story of the Women Who Helped Win World War II* (Atria Books, 2013).

17. Cuesta College, retrieved August 24, 2025, https://www.cuesta.edu/.

18. Cal Poly, retrieved August 24, 2025, https://www.calpoly.edu/.

19. Rotary, retrieved August 24, 2025, https://www.rotary.org/en.

20. M. Montanarella, A. Agarwal, and B. Moon, "Peripherally Inserted Central Catheter," *National Library of Medicine*, retrieved August 24, 2025, https://www.ncbi.nlm.nih.gov/books/NBK573064/.

21. "Nurse Ratched," *Wikipedia*, May 26, 2025, https://en.wikipedia.org/wiki/Nurse_Ratched.

22. University of California at San Francisco, "Lung Health Center," retrieved August 24, 2025, https://www.ucsfhealth.org/clinics/lung-health-center-at-parnassus.

23. POLST California, "California POLST Form," retrieved August 24, 2025, https://capolst.org/polst-for-healthcare-providers/forms/.

24. US Centers for Disease Control and Prevention, "About Necrotizing Fasciitis," retrieved August 24,

2025, https://www.cdc.gov/group-a-strep/about/ necrotizing-fasciitis.html.

25. "Quotes," *Goodreads*, retrieved August 24, 2025, https://www.goodreads.com/quotes/11988290-a-healthy-man-wants-a-thousand-things-a-sick-man.

26. Johns Hopkins Carey Business School, "Flexible MBA Specialization in Leadership," retrieved August 24, 2025, https://carey.jhu.edu/programs/flexible-mba/leadership.

27. Compassus, "What Is the We Honor Veterans Program?" retrieved August 24, 2025, https://www.compassus.com/for-caregivers/what-is-the-we-honor-veterans-program/.

28. Sharp HealthCare, "Sharp Allison DeRose Rehabilitation Center," retrieved August 24, 2025, https://www.sharp.com/locations/sharp-allison-derose-rehabilitation-center.

29. "Story of the Engine that Thought It Could, (1906, January 1)," *Wikisource*. https://en.wikisource.org/wiki/Story_of_the_Engine_that_Thought_It_Could.

30. Leading Age, "11th Hour Program Brings the Power of Connection to Those at the End of Life," May 24, 2024, https://leadingage.org/11th-hour-program-brings-the-power-of-connection-to-those-at-the-end-of-life/.

31. "Holocaust: Definition, Remembrance, and Meaning," *History*, retrieved August 24, 2025, https://www.history.com/articles/the-holocaust.

32. "God Bless America," *Wikipedia*, August 16, 2025, https://en.wikipedia.org/wiki/God_Bless_America.

33. Parkinson's Foundation, "Dementia with Lewy Bodies," retrieved August 24, 2025, https://www.parkinson.org/understanding-parkinsons/non-movement-symptoms/dementia/lewy-bodies.

34. R. W. Emerson, "To Laugh Often and Much," *All Poetry*, retrieved August 24, 2025, https://allpoetry.com/poem/14327880-To-Laugh-Often-And-Much-by-Ralph-Waldo-Emerson.

35. *Jay's Heart Podcast*, Spotify, https://creators.spotify.com/pod/profile/jaysheart/episodes/Intro-to-End-of-Life-e2celn9/a-aalonk3.

36. B. Gijsbertsen and J. Kremer, J. "We All Want to Die in Peace - So Why Don't We?" *BMJ Supportive and Palliative Care* 11, no. 3 (2020): 318–321, https://doi.org/DOI: 10.1136/bmjspcare-2019-002060.

37. M. Choudry and L. Ganti, "Exploration of the Motivational Factors that Influence the Maintenance of Health," *Health Psychology* Research, 2024, https://doi.org/ 10.52965/001c.115356.

38. U. Marusic, et al., "Nonuniform Loss of Muscle Strength and Atrophy during Bed Rest: A Systematic Review," *Journal of Applied Physiology* (2021), https://doi.org/ 10.1152/japplphysiol.00363.2020.

39. R. Epstein, R. and M. Krasner, "Physician Resilience: What It Means, Why It Matters, and How to Promote It," *Academic Medicine: Journal of the Association of American Medical Colleges* 88, no. 3 (2013): 301–303, https://doi.org/DOI: 10.1097/ACM.0b013e318280cff0.

About the Authors

Diane Wintz, MD, FACS, is the owner of Jay's Heart, which was formed in August 2023 as a legacy to her dad, Jay Schwartz, and his journey through heart disease and the transition to palliative care at the end of his life. This company prioritizes independence and quality of life during the medical journey, helping people to understand information and become educated on their options.

Dr. Wintz is board-certified in general surgery and surgical critical care, having completed her residency and fellowship at the University of Texas Health Science Center in Houston, Texas. She cares for injured patients through her hospital practice in California. She is the medical director for trauma and a new program called Generational Health, which is a multidisciplinary health-care package for hospitalized older adults who want to maintain independence and cognition. Dr. Wintz's outcomes research on trauma mentorship and geriatric trauma has been nationally recognized, with several podium presentations at the World Trauma Congress and the American Association for the Surgery of Trauma. She presented "Geriatric Trauma: Building a Program from the Ground Up" at a Society of Trauma Nurses webinar in 2023. She is a member of the standards and verification committee for geriatric surgery with the American College of Surgeons (ACS). Dr. Wintz championed the creation of a geriatric center of excellence at Sharp Memorial Hospital, in part due to high geriatric volume in the trauma population. This has resulted in tremendous gains for the geriatric trauma population, as well as a workshop and a Pecha Kucha at the Institute for Healthcare Improvement's annual summit and publication in the *Journal of Trauma and Acute Care Surgery* showing decreased length of stay, mortality, delirium, and time to mobilization. Her team recorded several nationally syndicated podcasts for ACS, Geriatric Emergency Department Collaborative, and Fierce DEI. The program achieved geriatric surgery verification, level one status, through the ACS in 2024, making Sharp Memorial Hospital the first facility in Southern California to achieve this designation.

Dr. Wintz's main interest is to guide patients and their families through some of the toughest parts of end-of-life care.

Kelly Wright, MSN, MBA, RN, CHPN, OCN, is a registered nurse and coordinator for medical navigation services at Jay's Heart. Wright has board certification in oncology, hospice, and palliative care. She fosters the mission and vision of Jay's Heart by providing the best care for people in need through educating, identifying what matters most, and ensuring adequate resources are in place. She works closely with the Jay's Heart team, provides leadership to health-care professionals, and collaborates with experts to provide excellent care coordination for individuals and communities.

Wright is the nurse manager for Generational Health and Advanced Illness Management (AIM) at Sharp Memorial Hospital in San Diego, California. She is a transformational leader in health care, and focuses on revolutionizing the experience for older adults by honoring their individual wishes. She began her career in oncology, where her leadership qualities led to her promotion to manager of the AIM team through peer nomination. Her leadership journey continued when she was promoted by the chief nursing officer to lead the development of the Generational Health team, addressing the unique needs of older adults including surgical patients, healthy aging patients, and those transitioning to end-of-life care. Wright has developed programs, fostered relationships with administration, and reported quantifiable improvements while supporting colleagues in their new roles. Her nursing team engages with over five thousand patients annually, focusing on establishing code status, goals of care, surgical risk assessment, and vulnerability screening. Wright has been a podium presenter at prestigious conferences including the American College of Surgeons Quality and Safety Conference, the European nursing conference in Dublin, Ireland, and the American Geriatrics Society Presidential Abstract competition. She is instrumental in educating health-care professionals on end-of-life discussions, palliative care philosophy, and incorporating compassion into care plans.